Reimagining Men's Cancers

Praise for
Reimagining Men's Cancers

"The illnesses of famous patients receive enormous attention from the media and serve as touchstones for patients and families dealing with similar conditions. They also can help vulnerable patients avoid being tricked by hoaxes, such as the unorthodox anticancer regimen that may have even accelerated Steve McQueen's death from mesothelioma. By taking a series of famous cancer cases and looking at the actual information being received by the public, Doctors Boguski and Berman are furthering the important process of ascertaining exactly what these episodes teach us."

—**Barron H. Lerner, MD, PhD,** Professor of Medicine and Population Health, Division of Medical Ethics, New York University School of Medicine, New York Langone Medical Center and author, *When Illness Goes Public: Celebrity Patients and How We Look at Medicine* (Johns Hopkins University Press 2006)

"As an educator striving to effectively convey key points in a lecture, I find including a celebrity facet with other examples makes it easier for our students, trainees, and faculty to work through very complex concepts in a fun way. Celebrity Diagnosis provides credible information about health conditions and diagnoses for many popular figures today. I am able to use the resource in a professional capacity within the library as well in my courses and workshops on various topics related to genomic medicine and biomedical research."

—**Kristi L. Holmes, PhD,** Director, Galter Health Sciences Library at Northwestern University, Feinberg School of Medicine

"You have demonstrated that the relationship between celebrity health conditions and consumer search behavior online has considerable potential for developing teachable moments for the advancement of public health. This is a highly innovative project with potentially big impact."

—**Nan M. Laird, PhD,** Harvey V. Fineberg Professor of Biostatistics, Harvard School of Public Health

"Media coverage of celebrities contains little material that conveys useful health information. This is a missed opportunity that can and should be addressed."

—Dr. Katherine Smith, Johns Hopkins Bloomberg
School of Public Health

"*MedPage Today* found that since launching Celebrity Diagnosis on our site, page views have risen faster than any other blog we carry. We believe it's because celebrities attract attention as a jump-off point to educate. You have found a unique niche."

—Robert Stern, Advisory Board, *Everyday Health*,
former CEO, *MedPage Today*

"I must admit that using celebrity diagnoses as a platform for a book on cancer took me off guard, but then I read the manuscript—accurate, clear, useful information that the average person will read and understand, while realizing that some of their favorite celebrities have been through the same thing. If you or a loved one has been diagnosed with cancer or is at high risk, this book is for you."

—Ellen T. Matloff, MS, President and CEO of MyGeneCounsel,
founder and former director, Cancer Genetic Counseling
Program, Yale School of Medicine

Reimagining *Men's* Cancers

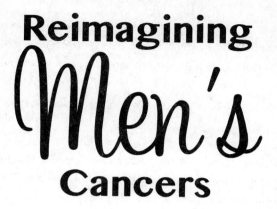

The Celebrity Diagnosis® Guide to Personalized Treatment and Prevention

Mark S. Boguski, MD, PhD, FCAP,
Michele R. Berman, MD,
and David Tabatsky

Health Communications, Inc.
Deerfield Beach, Florida

www.hcibooks.com

**Library of Congress Cataloging-in-Publication Data
is available through the Library of Congress**

© 2016 Mark S. Boguski, MD, PhD, FCAP, Michele R. Berman, MD, and David Tabatsky

ISBN-13: 978-07573-1955-6 (Paperback)
ISBN-10: 07573-1955-6 (Paperback)
ISBN-13: 978-07573-1956-3 (ePub)
ISBN-10: 07573-1956-4 (ePub)

Publisher: Health Communications, Inc.
    3201 S.W. 15th Street
    Deerfield Beach, FL 33442–8190

Cover design by Larissa Hise Henoch
Interior design and formatting by Lawna Patterson Oldfield

Contents

Acknowledgments

We launched *CelebrityDiagnosis.com* in 2008 with a mission to provide a dynamic collection of Teachable Moments in Medicine® to increase health awareness and medical knowledge by reporting on common diseases affecting uncommon people and the lessons these cases can provide for all of us.

Early inspiration for this work came from Barron Lerner, MD, PhD, and his book, *When Illness Goes Public: Celebrity Patients and How We Look at Medicine.* We thank Dr. Lerner for his early encouragement and continuing support.

Two other early supporters were Robert Stern, former CEO of *MedPage Today,* who first brought our work to the attention of healthcare professionals, and Helen Osborne, author of *Health Literacy from A To Z: Practical Ways to Communicate Your Health Message,* who increased awareness of our work through her *Health Literacy Out Loud* podcasts.

When Dr. Nan Laird of the Harvard T. H. Chan School of Public Health learned about our venture into celebrity health journalism, she initially counseled us to keep our day jobs. We thank her for advice and steadfast support, particularly in applying for grant funding from NIH.

Kirsten Ostherr, PhD, MPH, recognized the unique pedagogical value of our work and incorporated it into her popular course on *Medicine & Media* at Rice University. We thank Professor Ostherr and her students for their contributions to our mission.

Joel Aronowitz, MD, of the Breast Preservation Foundation, and Stephanie Holvick, RN, of *RNFaces.com*, educated us about the aesthetic and psychological dimensions of treating and recovering from cancer. We thank them for allowing us to interview them for our book.

Michael Misialek, MD, at Newton-Wellesley Hospital, Ellen Matloff, MS, CGC, at *MyGeneCounsel.com*, and Georgia Hurst, at *www.IhaveLynchSyndrome.com*, expended considerable time and effort in reviewing the medical content of our book and for this we are very grateful. Although every effort has been made to ensure that the information was correct and up to date at press time, any errors or omissions are the responsibility of the authors.

Margaret Foti, PhD, MD, (hc) of the American Association for Cancer Research has been a friend and colleague for more than twenty years. We share a passion for educating people about cancer and we thank her for her continuing friendship and sponsorship of our work.

Dr. Paul Laffer has been a valued adviser and enthusiastic supporter of our mission.

And, of course, we are grateful to Nancy Rosenfeld, our literary agent, for connecting us with HCI; Christine Belleris, Kim Weiss, and the entire team have been great to work with and we look forward to continuing our relationship with them as this series evolves.

We would be remiss not to acknowledge the celebrities included in this book who have made their stories available to the general public. Their willingness to help create these Teachable Moments in Medicine cannot be underestimated. We encourage other celebrities to also come forward and share their stories, as they play valuable roles in educating the public and inspiring them to take whatever preventative measures they can in maintaining good health.

David Tabatsky has been a phenomenal partner in this endeavor. His skill and experience are only matched by his warmth and humanity, and this project simply wouldn't have been possible without him. Thank you, David!

The final stages of book production competed for our attention with preparations for our daughter's wedding. We were able to pull off both by heeding Wilfred Arian Peterson's advice in *The Art of a Good Marriage*, including being flexible, patient, understanding and having a sense of humor.

—*Michele Berman and Mark Boguski*
Boston, MA

I would like to thank Michele and Mark for their lovely dispositions, friendship, and clearheaded approach to such a complicated subject. It's a total pleasure to work with them.

I'd also like to thank Nancy Rosenfeld, Christine Belleris and everyone at HCI for their commitment to this project.

Finally, may I acknowledge the wonderful people who have inspired the *My Journey* stories in both of these books. You inspire more people than you could ever imagine.

And to Dani, Bob, Jamie, Jan, Linn, and Rick—my love and gratitude.

—*David Tabatsky*
New York City

Introduction

Information is empowering, especially when it's dispensed in manageable doses. Reading about people coping with cancer—the same one you are dealing with—is not only educational and inspiring, it can save a life. Couple that with our fascination with celebrities and there is much we can learn from their experiences.

Celebrity cancer memoirs, including *The Time of My Life* by Patrick Swayze and Lisa Niemi Swayze (Atria 2010), *Resilience: Reflections on the Burdens and Gifts of Facing Life's Adversities* by Elizabeth Edwards (Broadway Books 2006), *Cancer Schmancer* by Fran Drescher (Grand Central Publishing 2002), *Time on Fire: My Comedy of Terrors* by Evan Handler (Little, Brown and Co. 1996, Argo-Navis 2012), provide readers with a "behind the scenes" look at how a famous person dealt with a cancer challenge that may be common to many of us. Not surprisingly, their struggles are essentially no different from any of ours.

It's no secret that celebrity information not only sells, it can educate people about many important issues—including cancer.

According to *USA Today*, when Katie Couric's colonoscopy was broadcast on live television, colonoscopy rates rose more than 20 percent. A similar reaction occurred in 2008 when Hall of Fame basketball player and NBA commentator Charles Barkley invited American television viewers to an on-air broadcast of his colonoscopy. Even Dr. Oz got in on the act, which created a noticeable spike in men's screenings for colon cancer. When Michael Douglas shared his throat cancer story, he taught us about the connection between human papillomavirus (HPV), oral sex, and head and neck cancers. Angelina Jolie's op-ed in the *New York Times*, detailing her genetic predisposition to breast and ovarian cancers and her subsequent decision to undergo a bilateral mastectomy, educated millions of people on the issue of genetic screening and preventive treatments and inspired them to take a proactive role in managing their own health.

Hamish Pringle, author of *Celebrity Sells* (John Wiley & Sons 2004) and former Director General of the Institute of Practitioners in Advertising, explains that "the role celebrities play in people's lives goes beyond a voyeuristic form of entertainment; they actually fulfill an extremely important research and development function for them as individuals and for society at large. People use celebrities as role models and guides."

That's what "infotainment" can do and what we hope *Reimagining Men's Cancer* exemplifies by dedicating itself to specific cancers affecting men and the people they love.

Because every twenty-three seconds someone in America is diagnosed with cancer, the number of people affected is continuing to grow and the data is not encouraging. The American Cancer Society estimates that nearly 2 million *new* patients will need treatment in the coming year. A recent World Cancer Report from the World Health Organization expects a 57 percent rise in cancer cases in the next twenty years.

Christopher Wild, director of the International Agency for Research on Cancer, says, "We cannot treat our way out of the cancer problem. More commitment to prevention and early detection is desperately needed in order to complement improved treatments and address the alarming rise in cancer burden globally."

The report says about half of all cancers are preventable and can be avoided if current medical knowledge is better delivered. The disease could be tackled by addressing lifestyle factors, such as smoking, alcohol consumption, diet, and exercise; adopting screening programs; or, in the case of infection-triggered cancers such as cervical and liver cancers, through vaccines. "The rise of cancer is a major obstacle to human development and well-being," Wild says. "Immediate action is needed to confront this human disaster."

This emphasis on prevention and early detection demonstrates the necessity and value of education. It is the key for anyone who might otherwise not pay attention to an epidemic that is likely to affect him or her or a loved one.

But a diagnosis of cancer is not—and does not have to be—an automatic death sentence. With advances in genomic (DNA) testing and diagnosis, we have learned that cancer—if detected early—can be managed just like many other chronic diseases or, in many cases, prevented through changes in diet, exercise, and general lifestyle.

That includes developing a sense of humor, which has proven time and time again to help everyone, from patients to doctors and especially those who can't figure out what to do or say when confronted with such a big challenge.

Consider the story of Jamile, a single father from Cincinnati, whose young daughter struggled to get accept his going bald as a result of his cancer treatment. One day, in an effort to lighten up the situation, he picked her up from school with three of his friends all wearing caps to make them appear bald while they serenaded Jamile's daughter and her classmates with a rousing and funny rendition of Willow Smith's hit song "Whip My Hair." She was delighted, as were her friends, and, from then on, being bald took on a whole new meaning for this child and her father.

In 2013, actress cancer survivor Christina Applegate told *womens healthmag.com*, "I laughed more in the hospital than I ever have in my life, making fun of all the weird things that were happening to me. My friends would walk in with this sad look, and I would throw something at them and say, 'Come on! This isn't the end of the world!'"

Herbie Mann, the legendary jazz musician who formed the Herbie Mann Prostate Cancer Awareness Music Foundation after being diagnosed in 1998 and gave concerts at which he offered free screening to all men in attendance between the ages of forty and seventy-five, shared similar sentiments. "When I first got cancer, after the initial shock and the fear and paranoia and crying and all that goes with cancer—that word means to most people ultimate death—I decided to see what I could do to take that negative and use it in a positive way."

This book is full of authentic and encouraging anecdotal evidence—from celebrities we have come to admire and trust as well as from "normal" people with valuable viewpoints of their own—who together offer us remarkably useful teachable moments that can educate and inspire and, in some cases, serve as life-saving cautionary tales.

Celebrity Diagnosis, the website we founded and launched in 2009, which is now featured as an integral part of the American Association for Cancer Research (AACR) Foundation website, combines celebrity health conditions (diagnosis, treatment, survivorship, etc.) with up-to-date medical information on common and uncommon cancers. By doing so, we have created numerous teachable moments in medicine, leading visitors to increase their health awareness and medical knowledge, which subsequently increases the likelihood of their considering early detection and preventive behavior.

"We have found from our own reporting on medical news," says Robert Stern, CEO of *MedPageToday*, a leading source of medical information online, "that nothing resonates with our professional clinician readers more than a celebrity illness because call volume to offices increases from patients when a celebrity is diagnosed. This provides a teachable moment for the physician to share with the patient."

The AACR, with its 35,000 members from around the globe,

making it the oldest and largest scientific organization in the world, agrees, and by featuring Celebrity Diagnosis it is now expanding its support of high-quality, innovative cancer research and education. Through its numerous publications and frequent conferences, the AACR works with a vast umbrella of cancer organizations, hospitals, and individuals.

Meanwhile, the pharmaceutical industry, with its mission to address unmet medical needs by developing new drugs, still takes ten to fifteen years at an average cost of $2.4 billion to sponsor the applied research, tech development, and regulatory requirements to develop a single new drug, which may or may not serve its intended purpose.

What about the needs of consumers for better access to existing medical knowledge and practices? Can increasing health awareness and providing scientific information lead to better use of existing resources, including prevention and early detection screening methods? Social media and mass market books can be valuable allies in the task to equip people with what is necessary to manage and improve their own health.

We certainly hope so. That's why our philosophy of Participatory Medicine is a lynchpin of Celebrity Diagnosis and a key to empowering people to partner with their doctors in taking responsibility for their healing.

The definition of a modern "e-patient" is to be *engaged, equipped,* and *empowered,* three integral qualities that form the foundation of our approach.

Dr. Katherine Smith of Johns Hopkins Bloomberg School of Public Health feels that traditional media coverage of celebrities contains little material that conveys useful health information, concluding that "media attention to such newsworthy events is a missed opportunity that can and should be addressed."

We agree. There seems to be a large missed opportunity to educate people about prevention and personal empowerment. That's why *Reimagining Men's Cancers* now exists—to inform, inspire, and ignite the appropriate action that is needed to live healthier lives. But you may ask, What does a famous person have to do with me? Studies of the power of celebrity to create teachable moments, such as those conducted by Professor Graeme Turner of the University of Queensland Centre for Critical and Cultural Studies, Hamish Pringle at the Institute of Practitioners of Advertising, and Robert Havighurst, PhD, author of *Human Development and Education*, suggest that the personal life experiences of individuals we admire and respect from popular culture can create teachable moments that may be vicarious at first but ultimately prove to be educational and, in some cases, lifesaving.

According to Mable Kinzie of the University of Virginia Curry School of Education, who has developed instructional design strategies for health behavior change, there is a five-step process to developing educational materials and making sure they resonate and connect, producing real results.

It begins with gaining attention by featuring famous people whose health has become a news item, and then providing information on specific conditions (in this case, men's cancers). It continues by guidance through clear and concise information about how a particular cancer exists and operates, as well as supplying anecdotal reports, interviews, and expert medical resources. When presented together, these enhance retention and stimulate appropriate social discourse that inevitably shares this knowledge with others.

For someone newly diagnosed with male-specific cancers, such as prostate, penile, and/or testicular—or for those suddenly thrust into the role of caregiver—the medical information provided here is easy to find and read, providing you with a comprehensive overview of the particular cancer's traits, warning signs, symptoms, diagnostic techniques, as well as prognoses and treatments, both traditional and alternative. This medical information is complemented by personal accounts and interviews from celebrities and non-celebrities who have been challenged by the same cancers.

For example, the chapter on prostate cancer begins with a view of basic anatomy; an overview of how we view this particular cancer today; signs, symptoms, and diagnosis; as well as scientific information on screening guidelines. You'll find a comprehensive survey of treatments, prevention, and short- and long-term forecasts.

Woven throughout the book are celebrity stories, both medical and anecdotal, from men, including Michael Douglas, Robert De Niro, Mandy Patinkin, Harry Belafonte, Lance Armstrong, and many others, as well as stories from men you may recognize as neighbors, colleagues, and friends.

Since scientific concepts such as DNA and the human genome have become commonplace through television shows like *CSI* and *Dr. Oz*, as well as other media like the *New York Times* and *Time* magazine, this vital information is now more accessible than ever and much better understood by the general public, enabling patients and caregivers to raise their level of interaction with their doctors.

We like to cite the Angelina Jolie Effect, which has caused curiosity about cancer and DNA/genetic testing to skyrocket, as more and more patients are asking to have their tumor genomes analyzed in order to select the right drug treatment for them.

When news of a celebrity being diagnosed with cancer goes public, physicians invariably see a sharp increase in the volume of calls to their offices and online search-engine traffic spikes regarding the specific disease or medical condition associated with that celebrity diagnosis.

We refer to this interface between health communication and pop culture as the Goody-Gaga Effect, which refers to the sudden increase in public interest in a specific disease or medical condition when it is associated with a celebrity. The Goody-Gaga Effect is named after the late British TV personality Jade Goody, whose battle with cervical cancer was followed daily in the UK, and Lady Gaga, who made her "borderline positive" lupus test public, prompting a huge spike in the attention and support given to that disease.

But when celebrities (or their publicists) talk about cancer or other medical issues, the results can be mixed. If they mistakenly publicize information that is confusing or contradictory to established medical protocols, they may cause harm. On the other hand, when they provide the public with an accurate, inside look at their situation, this can become a teachable moment and lives can be saved. Exploring examples of how this works is not only instructive and, in some cases entertaining, it colors the way we essentially view celebrity and the manners in which we might disseminate and digest life-altering information.

Brian L. Dyak, president and cofounder of the Entertainment Industries Council and the Entertainment and Media Communication Institute and the award-winning creator of the PRISM Awards (FX Networks) television special, is a pioneer of "edutainment," which promotes the power of celebrity to depict health issues. For over twenty-five years, Dyak has successfully constructed a bridge between the entertainment industry and health and social policy issues. His thoughts on the link between the entertainment industry and national health have inspired us to reach more people with the foundational information you will find in this book.

Unfortunately, cancer is not going away anytime soon but neither is our fascination with celebrities, especially when they—like any of us—become vulnerable. With this in mind, the need to educate and heal is clear. For the more than 230,000 men who are diagnosed with gender-specific cancers (prostate, penile, testicular, bladder, breast) each year in the United States—as well as for the loved ones and medical professionals who care for them—we hope this book will offer great benefits.

Barron Lerner, MD, Professor of Medicine and Public Health at Columbia University College of Physicians and Surgeons, demonstrates in his book *When Illness Goes Public: Celebrity Patients and How We Look at Medicine* how celebrities significantly influence public attitudes toward diseases and their treatments. Lerner concludes that celebrity cases can educate the public, create advocates for research and care on behalf of other people with the same disease, and even influence aspects of the professional training of physicians.

By exercising the powerful magic of storytelling, celebrities are capable of influencing people in a wide variety of ways. But they can do much more than move us emotionally. They can raise our awareness about cancer and, in many cases, even prompt their fans to become better informed and seek the preventive care and early diagnostic screening they need.

People in the public eye have the potential to provide teachable moments in medicine. We can learn from them, as we can from most anyone who has experienced cancer. Anyone who has been diagnosed and undergone treatment has something to offer. Anyone who has served as a personal caretaker has wisdom to share. And medical professionals of all stripes have much insight to offer.

Together, the anecdotes and experiences shared here in *Reimagining Men's Cancers* provide a substantial collection of cancer portraits, and, along with all of the comprehensive medical information, you should be able to find much of what you may need in order to understand what you are dealing with and to figure out how best to proceed. Most important, you will be better equipped to communicate effectively with your doctors, which should provide you the best-case scenario for making what can often be difficult choices.

Emmarie Truman, who was diagnosed with cancer as a teenager, was given a button one day while in a radiation room that read "Cancer Sucks." She agreed that this is the best way to look at it. "Cancer does suck," she said, "and the sooner you accept that, the sooner you can realize that no matter how much it sucks you have to deal with it and that you might as well deal with it with a smile."

This simple lesson is not to be overlooked. You will find that *Reimagining Men's Cancers* is full of them. By combining the inspiration of "average" patients and the power of celebrity stories with vital information about common and uncommon cancers, we hope that this book will help you become better informed as a patient and/or a patient advocate.

In his State of the Union address earlier this year, President Obama announced a new Moonshot to Cure Cancer campaign—the "Precision Medicine Initiative"—to eradicate cancer as soon as possible and was inspired, in part, by the tragic loss of Vice President Joe Biden's son Beau to cancer in 2015. Such a high-profile case can lead to increased awareness in the general public as well as launch renewed efforts on governmental and private institutional levels to prevent and eventually eradicate this disease.

In the chapters that follow, we'll explain why the time is ripe, as MD Anderson Cancer Center says, to "make cancer history" through the cutting-edge practice of precision medicine using sophisticated targeted treatments that attack the root causes of the disease.

Together, we can make a difference.

A Note on Resources and Celebrity Diagnosis

Throughout *Reimagining Men's Cancer*, we present relevant scientific data about each type of cancer discussed in a particular chapter. Because this book is not primarily intended to be a textbook for medical students/doctors but rather a guide and teaching tool for *anyone*, we have attempted to dose out the medical information in easy-to-read and appropriately digestible pieces that are manageable and satisfying.

Those seeking additional medical information/anecdotal stories about other celebrities with cancer can visit *www.celebritydiagnosis. com*.

A Note on Non-Celebrity Stories

In an effort to provide a comprehensive collection of patients and caregivers affected by men's cancers, we have selected from a wide assortment of anecdotes, blogs, interviews, and stories from men and women throughout the country. Each of the My Journey segments in this book represents an individualized composite of the many people we have been in contact with over the past several years.

1 A NEW MIND-SET:
Reimagining Cancer as a Manageable Chronic Illness

*The ultimate measure of a man is
not where he stands in moments of comfort
and convenience, but where he stands at
a time of challenge and controversy.*

—Dr. Martin Luther King Jr.

The Evolution of Cancer Treatment:
From Toxic "Weapons of Mass Destruction"
to Targeted Therapy

In 2008, legendary basketball player Kareem Abdul-Jabbar began experiencing frequent hot flashes and night sweats. Doctors found his blood clogged with white cells containing something called the Philadelphia chromosome, and his diagnosis was a type of leukemia called CML. If Mr. Abdul-Jabbar had been diagnosed with CML ten years earlier, in 1998, the next steps would have been a series of injections with toxic drugs similar in chemical composition to mustard gas, a World War I–era weapon of mass destruction, followed by irradiation of his entire body.

These treatments were meant to destroy DNA and the cancer cells along with it. But since DNA is present in all human cells, the chemotherapy and radiation couldn't discriminate between cancer cells and normal cells. That is why this type of therapy is plagued by toxic side effects. Many types of cancer, not just CML, were, and still are, treated with these chemicals and radiation, which we often refer to as weapons of mass destruction (WMDs).

So what changed the landscape in those ten years between 1998 and 2008? It was the introduction in 2001 of Gleevec, the first "magic bullet" cancer drug. Instead of offering treatment with a WMD cocktail, the twenty-first century war on cancer is now conducted with the medical equivalent of precision-guided smart munitions, similar in concept to smart bombs and precision-guided missiles. All of these weapons are designed to specifically target cancer cells and minimize collateral damage.

Kareem Abdul-Jabbar and the Magic Cancer Bullet

Mr. Abdul-Jabbar was treated with one of these targeted therapies —a little orange pill called imatinib, known commercially as Gleevec. These "magic cancer bullets" have now become the gold standard for treatment of CML and many other types of cancer, including skin (melanoma) and lung cancers. The U.S. Food and Drug Administration (FDA) now approves approximately three dozen additional targeted therapies similar to imatinib. Hundreds more are in development by drug companies.

According to the FDA, imatinib is now used to treat several types of leukemia and other cancers of the bone marrow. It is also used to treat gastrointestinal stromal tumors and a rare sarcoma.

The lesson of Gleevec is that once we understand the underlying cause of a cancer and can precisely diagnose it, this knowledge almost always extends to other cancers as well.

Dr. Francis Collins and Christopher Hitchens: The Language of God Meets Personalized Medicine

Dr. Francis Collins was the director of the Human Genome Project and is the current director of the National Institutes of Health (NIH). Dr. Collins is also an evangelical Christian who wrote a book about DNA, defining genes as *The Language of God.*

Dr. Collins often engaged in friendly debates about God's existence with author, journalist, and celebrated atheist Christopher Hitchens. When the sixty-year-old Mr. Hitchens was diagnosed with cancer of the esophagus in 2010, Dr. Collins reached out to his debate partner with the possibility of using advanced DNA techniques to analyze Hitchens's cancer and pick the right treatment, a process sometimes called personalized medicine.

The standard treatment for cancer of the esophagus is surgery, but Mr. Hitchens's cancer had already spread and was in its most advanced state: stage IV. As Mr. Hitchens dryly observed, "There is no stage V." Treatment for Mr. Hitchens's advanced cancer was similar to what a CML patient would have received in 1998—chemical and radiation WMDs.

But Dr. Collins and his colleagues made a startling discovery in Hitchens's tumor's DNA. They identified a "misprint" that might respond to the same drug that turned Kareem Abdul-Jabbar's cancer into a manageable chronic illness: imatinib (Gleevec).

Today, in an increasing number of cases, cancer is being transformed from a deadly disease into a manageable chronic illness. This reimagining of cancer is made possible by research advances that allow more precise diagnosis and personalized treatment. In the near future, new technologies will enable detection and diagnosis of cancer in a drop of blood rather than in a piece of the cancer surgically removed from a patient.

―――――――――――― **MY JOURNEY** ――――――――――――

Over a span of several years, I was diagnosed four separate times with cancer. It became routine to see people taken back when they heard my story. They were usually tongue-tied, especially when I said, "I'm trying out a few different cancers and I hope to find one I really like." Their reactions were amazing, and it suggests that cancer may very well be something we can actually live with—maybe even, like my wife says, "live long and prosper."

Jerry (Roanoke, Virginia)

Grading and Staging Tumors

After a diagnosis of cancer, but *before* treatment begins, a patient almost always goes through a process called grading and staging that determines the type(s) of treatment, the intensity of these treatments, and how long they will have to continue.

This grading and staging process is often called a workup, described here in detail.

What Is My Grade and Who Does the Grading?

Just when you thought your school days were a distant memory in your rearview mirror, that you were done being evaluated and assigned numbers and letters for some accomplishment or skill, the scientific facts of a cancer diagnosis can slingshot you right back to the days of being graded and placed on a level of someone else's ladder.

You might ask, "What are the rungs of a cancer ladder, and is it better to be high or low?"

First, let's look at how a tumor is graded. Using a microscope to examine very thin slices of a cancer from a biopsy specimen that have been stained with pink and purple dyes, a specialist doctor, called a surgical pathologist, compares these slices with normal, noncancerous tissue and assesses how far the tumor cells and their "architecture" have deviated from their normal appearance.

Unlike in school, where a higher grade is usually preferred, tumor grades are just the opposite: the lower the better.

There are different grading systems for different types of cancer. For example, the grading of prostate cancer (Chapter 2) is done using the Gleason grading scale, or score. But, in general, tumors are graded on this type of scale:

GX: Grade cannot be assessed (undetermined grade)
G1: Well differentiated (low grade)
G2: Moderately differentiated (intermediate grade)
G3: Poorly differentiated (high grade)
G4: Undifferentiated (high grade)

Low-grade tumors are described as well differentiated because they clearly resemble the normal tissue (for example, prostate glands) in which the tumor arose. High-grade tumors look undifferentiated, meaning that the tumor cells and architecture barely resemble, if at all, the normal tissue they came from.

More than a century ago, doctors discovered that a tumor's grade was a good predictor of its tenacity and aggressiveness. In other words, the higher the grade, the more difficult it was to treat the cancer, which meant a less favorable prognosis for the patient. Unfortunately, the same holds true today, but with more sophisticated, effective treatment options, a patient's prognosis does not necessarily mean the same thing now as it did back then.

Meet Your Pathologist—Or Not

The medical process of a pathology diagnosis is the gold standard by which cancer is diagnosed and upon which treatment plans are based. The specialist who performs this diagnosis is called a pathologist. Unfortunately, he or she is often the only member of a care team—and the most important doctor—the patient will probably *never* meet.

Pathologists are medical doctors who spend an additional four to five years after medical school learning the field of laboratory medicine. Television shows like *CSI* or *Body of Proof* depict pathologists as performing autopsies to help police and prosecutors determine the manner and cause of death. But these doctors are forensic pathologists or medical examiners and have nothing to do with the routine diagnosis of cancer for patient care.

Most pathologists spend their time detecting and analyzing tissue biopsies, blood samples, urine samples, and other types of specimens collected from living patients. It's the job of the pathologist to diagnose whether the biopsy specimen represents, for example, prostate cancer or something else, such as an infection (prostatitis) or BPH (benign prostatic hypertrophy). It's also the pathologist's job to perform and analyze blood tests, such as PSA (Chapter 2), that are used for cancer screening, detection, response to treatments, and recurrence.

Although many pathologists don't routinely interact directly with patients, this doesn't mean that the patient can't ask to meet or talk with the pathologist whose expertise is one of the most critical factors in a cancer patient's prognosis and care.

One extremely important step in the process that can affect the accuracy of the pathologic diagnosis is how the patient's tissue specimen is handled and processed during the time between its surgical removal and its arrival in the pathology lab. The details of tissue processing and transport are called preanalytic variables. If certain strict protocols are not followed, this process can result in a missed or incorrect diagnosis.

> ### NOTE to PATIENT:
> We recommend that if and when you become a patient and are asked to sign a consent form for a biopsy or other type of surgery, you inquire about which pathologist will be responsible for handling your specimen and whether there are any special protocols for processing your tissue based on the type of cancer you are suspected of having.

In case of unexpected findings at the time of surgery, your pathologist may be called to the operating room to consult with your surgeon in determining how the specimen should be handled. Therefore, it is essential that you speak up about these matters. Once again, this is a situation where assuming personal responsibility is in your best interest.

This is also because pathology, like many other sciences, does not always yield perfectly accurate results. While the practice of pathology relies on science, it also involves human judgment and experience, meaning mistakes can be made that may result in an incorrect or misleading diagnosis.

Last year, The Johns Hopkins Hospital in Baltimore reviewed tissue samples from 6,000 cancer patients nationwide and found one out of every seventy-one cases was misdiagnosed. In one case, emblematic of many they discovered, a biopsy was labeled cancerous when in fact it was not. They also found incorrect classifications in up to one out of five cases.

This type of error in judgment—in how fast or how far the cancer had spread—can significantly affect a patient's prognosis and care.

Dr. Jonathan Epstein of The Johns Hopkins Hospital concurs. "That can change whether a patient gets no treatment versus surgery versus radiation, and if they get surgery or radiation, which type."

According to this study and others, errors can be made in any biopsy, but they are found most often in tissue samples from the skin, prostate, breast, and female reproductive tract.

According to Dr. Leonard Zwelling of the MD Anderson Cancer Center in Houston, "We really still make the diagnosis pretty much the way we did for the last fifty years. It has to come down to looking at a piece of the tumor on a slide by a pathologist."

> **NOTE to PATIENT:**
> Get a second opinion from an expert pathologist.

Your pathologist's report is part of your medical record, and it is your right to obtain a copy of this report. Sometimes you may also want to obtain a second opinion from another pathologist with special expertise in your type of cancer.

Who and What Determines My Stage?

Unlike tumor grading, which is done with a microscope and the expertise of your pathologist, staging is a more complex process conducted by at least three doctors: an oncologist, a surgeon, and a medical imaging specialist, called a radiologist.

The goal of a staging workup is to accurately determine how far and where a cancer has spread.

Different types of cancer have different patterns of spread, largely based on your body's anatomy and drainage systems. These predictable patterns inform your doctors on where and how to focus their staging and, ultimately, their treatment efforts.

Staging your cancer has several important functions: It helps your doctor plan your treatment, assess your prognosis, and evaluate the results of your treatment. It can also play a role in determining if you qualify for participation in clinical research trials of new treatments.

Staging also helps medical researchers and public health officials exchange information about how different cancers affect different patients. It provides a common language for comparing the effectiveness of different treatments and planning effective screening methods and recommendations for population health.

Staging can be done through either surgery or imaging technologies, such as X-ray, CT, MRI, ultrasound, and a combination called PET/CT, which measures both the location of the tumor and the extent to which it is metabolically active.

Defining the Five Stages of Cancer

It is helpful to define the five stages of cancer.

Stage 0: Carcinoma *in situ* is an early cancer or precancer present only in the layer of cells where it began.

Stage I: The tumor is limited to the organ in which it formed.

Stage II: The tumor is more extensive but still limited to its organ of origin.

Stage III: The tumor has spread beyond its organ to adjacent tissues or is present in regional lymph nodes.

Stage IV: The tumor has metastasized (spread) to distant sites in the body.

Rasheen Davis, author of *The Chemo Room: My Journey Through Fear, Hope and Survival*, found out that staging is one of the most important numbers in a patient's life. It helps the doctor make a prognosis and plan appropriate treatment. Staging helps healthcare providers and researchers exchange information about patients. It also provides a common terminology to evaluate treatment results.

"Like a golfer," Rasheen says, "you want your score to be low, like I. Never IV."

TNM and the Logic of Cancer Progression

Cancer spreads locally along the path of least resistance from the primary site of the tumor (T). It also spreads to lymph nodes (N) that drain the organ or part of the body where the primary tumor is located. The lymph node closest to the tumor is called the sentinel node.

Cancer metastasizes (M) to distant organs or parts of the body through the blood stream.

Professor Pierre Denoix, a French surgeon, first developed the TNM system between 1943 and 1952. It has been further developed and maintained by the Union of International Cancer Control (UICC) and is the international standard for the staging of most solid tumors.

TMN letters are presented with numbers that indicate the progression of the cancer.

- T1, T2, T3, and T4 indicate increases in size or extent of a tumor.
- N1, N2, and N3 indicate the extent of spread to regional lymph nodes.
- M0 and M1 indicate the absence or presence of distant metastases, respectively.

Sometimes an X is used instead of a number, indicating that the tumor could not be assessed, which means the pathologist could not find any lymph nodes (NX) in the tumor specimen.

For many cancers, TNM combinations correspond to one of five stages. Criteria for stages differ for different cancer types, and you will find them described in subsequent chapters devoted to specific cancer types.

Crucial Questions for Your Doctor

For the more than 235,000 men diagnosed each year with new cases of prostate, breast, testicular, and penile cancers, there are a host of crucial questions they should ask their doctor. Our friends at *www. surviveit.org* suggest the following:

- Exactly what type of cancer do I have?
- What stage is my cancer in, and how does that affect my options?
- Is there any further testing available to better diagnose my cancer?
- Was my biopsy analyzed for any specific gene mutation(s)?
- Can further gene mutation testing diagnose my cancer more specifically?
- Should I see a certified genetic counselor to determine if my cancer is hereditary?
- If the gene mutation testing is negative, what treatment options are available?
- What do you recommend and why, and where can I learn more about this type of treatment?
- What risks or side effects are there to the treatment(s) you suggest?
- How is the treatment likely to help, and when will we know if it's working?
- What is the five-year survival rate for my specific stage and condition?
- Can you put me in contact with someone you treated with this treatment plan?

- Are there any clinical trials I should consider?
- Who is researching my type of cancer, and should I seek a second opinion from them?
- If they offer a targeted treatment plan or clinical trial, will you collaborate with them?
- How do you recommend I share my hopes and expectations with my family?
- What should I do to be ready for my next phase of treatment?

Once you've asked these questions, hopefully your doctors, nurses, and social workers will be asking appropriate questions of you. After all, they are human, too, and dealing with patients full time can be a humbling reminder of their own fragility.

"Those of us who work in oncology make a pact with the gods," says Hester Hill Schnipper, LICSW, BCD, OSW-C, chief of oncology social work at Beth Israel Deaconess Medical Center in Boston. "If we devote our lives to taking care of others, our own lives, and those of people whom we love, will be protected. Intellectually, we know that it's not so, but in our hearts, the contract is sealed."

The effects of cancer challenge the humanity of patients *and* medical professionals. That's why effective communication in both directions is essential to everyone's good health.

MY JOURNEY

After being diagnosed and working out a treatment plan with my oncologist, I went to buy the medicine I'd been prescribed. I was trying to pretend that it was just like getting an antibiotic for a normal infection. But my pharmacist recognized my anxiety and gave me some wise advice.

"One of the most important things to remember in the months ahead is what's between your ears," he said. "Your mind-set will play a big part in how you deal with this whole process."

I couldn't thank him enough. Between my doctor's positivity and my pharmacist spelling out for me the importance of maintaining a positive attitude, I've been constantly reminded to be grateful for each day and the people who make them valuable.

Taylor (Columbus, Ohio)

How Do I Explain It?

A diagnosis of cancer is a lot for anyone to digest, to say the least. When taking in and trying to process an onslaught of new information—let alone all the emotions that come with it—any previous experience with being sick, or taking care of someone who is, makes little to no difference.

And when you must explain your condition to others in your life—family, friends, colleagues, and neighbors—the task can be daunting. That's why having the right information is so essential—to help you understand what you're going through and to make it easier to communicate all of it with the important people in your life.

So whether it's prostate cancer or any of the other cancers that are gender specific to a man, we encourage you to be patient and keep reading, because you will find much of what you will need to know—and ask your medical team about—as you proceed through this journey.

KEY POINTS TO REMEMBER

✓ Reimagining cancer is made possible by research advances.

✓ Precision diagnoses and targeted treatments allow us to treat many cancers more effectively and with fewer side effects than in the past.

✓ Grading and staging of cancer are essential parts of the diagnostic process (the workup) and will provide important information on your prognosis and guide your treatment.

✓ Ask your doctor seventeen crucial questions.

✓ Your attitude plays a big part in how you deal with this entire process.

WHAT CANCER CANNOT DO

Cancer is so limited . . .
It cannot cripple love.

2 SILENT KILLER OR MANAGEABLE ILLNESS? What You Need to Know About Prostate Cancer

Oh, my friend, it's not what
they take away from you that counts.
It's what you do with what you have left.

—Hubert Humphrey, after cancer surgery in 1978

Becoming the Rule, Not the Exception

In 1934, Dr. Arnold Rice Rich, a pathologist at the Johns Hopkins Medical School in Baltimore, Maryland, made an astounding discovery. Based on the autopsies of 292 men over the age of fifty, Dr. Rich found cancer in the prostate glands of 14 percent of these men. These cancers had not been detected prior to their deaths—all of which were due to other causes.

Dr. Rich described these cancers as "occult," meaning "hidden from view." When he published his observations a year later, they were greeted with disbelief and largely forgotten.

In 1954, Dr. L. M. Franks, one of Rich's original disbelievers, delivered a lecture at the Royal College of Surgeons of England, reversing his previous position, as he had become convinced of the validity of Dr. Rich's work.

Dr. Franks called these prostate tumors "latent cancers." He believed that after the cancers reached a certain stage of development, further growth stopped and the tumors remained latent for a long period of time, quite often long enough that the affected men died of an unrelated condition.

But Dr. Franks disagreed with Dr. Rich about one aspect of these latent cancers. He felt that Dr. Rich's estimate of 14 percent of men was much too low. He cited other studies showing that up to 44 percent of men had these latent or occult cancers in their prostate glands.

Let's fast-forward to 2012, when a study[1] from the Harvard School of Public Health determined that men who have been diagnosed with prostate cancer are more likely to die from largely preventable conditions, such as heart disease, than from prostate cancer. In fact, recent studies from 2013 show that hidden prostate cancers are present in 40 percent of men ages sixty and older and in 60 percent of men who are over the age of eighty.

Prostate cancer is the most common non-skin cancer in America, affecting one out of every six men during their lifetimes. Nearly 3 million men are currently living in the United States with prostate cancer, and approximately 221,000 new cases are diagnosed each year. About

---

1. M.M. Epstein, G. Edgren, J.R. Rider, L.A. Mucci, and H.O. Adami, "Temporal trends in cause of death among Swedish and US men with prostate cancer." *Journal of the National Cancer Institute* 2012 (September 5, 2012); 104 (17):1335–42.

28,000 men die as a result of prostate cancer every year, but this is less than 1 percent of the 3 million men currently living with the disease.

According to most medical experts today, if a man lives long enough, he is more likely to die *with* prostate cancer than *from* prostate cancer.

Basic Anatomy and Function

The prostate is a walnut-sized gland that weighs about one ounce and lies just below the bladder and in front of a man's rectum. Its function is to add fluid to support and nourish sperm, because together, prostate fluid plus sperm equals semen.

The urethra, the tube through which urine flows from the bladder to the penis, passes through the prostate. When a man has an orgasm, muscle fibers surrounding prostate glands push prostate fluid, combined with sperm, from the testicles, into the urethra, and out through the tip of the penis. This is what naturally occurs during ejaculation.

The prostate gland is covered in a layer of connective tissue called a capsule. The internal structure of the prostate gland is made up of different types of cells, including the following:

- *Acini*: These are tiny glands made up of cells that produce the fluid portion of semen.
- *Muscle cells*: These control urine flow and ejaculation.
- *Fibrous cells*: These provide the supportive structure of the gland.

The prostate gland has three zones: peripheral, transition, and central.

The peripheral zone is closest to the rectum and can be felt by a physician during a digital rectal examination (DRE). Approximately 75 percent of prostate tumors are located in the peripheral zone.

The transition zone is in the midsection of the prostate, surrounding the urethra. Until the age of forty, it makes up about 20 percent

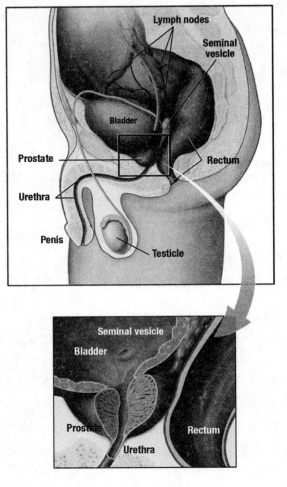

The Prostate
Source: National Cancer Institute

of the gland. However, as a man ages, the transition zone begins to enlarge, and ultimately becomes the largest zone of the prostate.

The central zone lies in front of the transition zone, farthest from the rectum, and cannot be felt on a DRE.

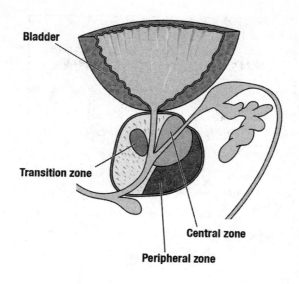

Zones of the Prostate
Source: Peter Lamb (through *123rf.com*)

——————— MY JOURNEY ———————

I didn't even know I had a prostate until my wife told me I should get it checked out once I turned fifty. At first, I ignored her, and a bunch of my friends were basically doing the same thing with their wives. I mean, we love these women in our lives, but I'm not big on seeing doctors or having anybody poke me for no good reason. But when my best friend was diagnosed with prostate cancer, I figured all bets are off, so I agreed to go to my doctor.

So far, so good, one year at a time. I'll keep checking because my wife has me convinced that it's the right thing to do. Thank God I'm married or I'd probably be dead. But that's for a lot of reasons!

Max (Miami, Florida)

How the Prostate Ages (and BPH)

A man's prostate goes through two main growth periods during his life. The first phase occurs early in puberty, when the prostate doubles in size. The second phase of growth begins around age twenty-five and continues during most of a man's life. Benign prostatic hyperplasia (BPH) often occurs during the second growth phase and affects about 50 percent of men between the ages of fifty-one and sixty and up to 90 percent of men older than eighty.

As the prostate enlarges, the gland presses against the urethra and pinches it. The bladder wall becomes thicker. Eventually, the bladder may weaken and lose its ability to empty completely, leaving some urine in the bladder. The narrowing of the urethra and urinary retention—the inability to empty the bladder completely—cause many of the problems associated with BPH.

But BPH is *not* cancer. The letter *B* stands for "benign." However, since some of the signs and symptoms of prostate cancer can also occur in patients with BPH, it's an important condition to know about. Your doctor can advise you on available treatments.

The Blessing and the Curse of PSA Testing

In the late 1960s and early 1970s, medical researchers were searching for proteins that were present only in the prostate gland and no other organs or tissues of the body. If such a protein could be identified, it might possibly be important as a target for treatment or as a biomarker for the presence of prostate cancer.

At the time, the typical approach for identifying such a protein was to put samples of the human prostate gland in a blender to liquefy the tissue and then inject some of this tissue extract into a rabbit. The rabbit's immune system would then make antibodies against the human proteins, which are called antigens. These antihuman, rabbit antibodies could then be used to study potential targets or biomarkers in human tissues and fluids, such as prostate biopsies and blood.

A number of scientists, including Dr. Richard Ablin and Dr. Ming Chu, succeeded in identifying a protein that was present only in prostate tissue and called it prostate specific antigen, better known today as PSA. Apart from being specific to prostate tissue, it also became clear that the normal, biological function of PSA is to break down other proteins in seminal fluid to make it more liquid. PSA's use as a biomarker or diagnostic test is entirely unrelated to its normal function in the prostate gland and the creation of seminal fluid.

PSA is not specific for cancer, but cancer cells retain the ability to make PSA and it leaks into the bloodstream from tumors. Dr. Chu and his colleagues at Roswell Park Cancer Institute in Buffalo, New York, used this fact to devise a test to measure PSA in the blood, and in 1984 they were awarded a U.S. patent. Just two years later, the U.S. Food and Drug Administration (FDA) approved the PSA test as a way to monitor treatment response and disease recurrence in patients who had already been diagnosed with prostate cancer. This test has been a great blessing to patients and their doctors and is still in use today for managing patients with prostate cancer.

In 1994, the FDA approved PSA testing as a way to screen men for early detection of prostate cancer during their annual physical exams, even if they have no signs or symptoms of the disease. Since then, more than a billion PSA tests have been performed.

But eventually, problems with overdiagnosis and overtreatment have become a concern. As we said before, PSA is not specific for cancer; blood levels of PSA can be elevated by noncancerous conditions, such as infection or inflammation (prostatitis) and BPH. Many medical authorities have come to the conclusion that population screening using PSA leads to unnecessary biopsies, overdiagnosis, and overtreatment of low-grade, indolent tumors that would never otherwise affect the health or lifespan of the patient.

As discussed in Chapter 10, based on a harm-benefit analysis, the U.S. Preventive Services Task Force (USPSTF) recommended in 2012 against using PSA as a screening test for prostate cancer. There may still be some circumstances in which your doctor feels that PSA testing is important—for example, if you have a family history of prostate cancer or you have an abnormal DRE or you are suffering from certain symptoms. But for most men, the PSA test should no longer be routinely used as part of their annual checkups.

Robert De Niro:
An Unexpected Role to Play

Two-time Academy Award–winning actor Robert De Niro is known for playing tough guys in films such as *Raging Bull, Taxi Driver*, and *The Godfather Part II*. But in 2003, at the age of sixty, De Niro had to take on perhaps his toughest real-life role: that of a prostate cancer patient. According to his publicist, Stan Rosenfield, "The condition was detected at an early stage because of regular checkups, a result of his proactive personal healthcare program."

Between the early detection and De Niro's excellent physical condition, his doctors anticipated a full recovery. After surgery and treatment at New York's Memorial Sloan-Kettering Cancer Center, they were proven correct, and De Niro's career has continued to flourish both in films and his philanthropic work. And in 2011, at age sixty-eight, De Niro became a father for the sixth time, when his daughter Helen Grace Hightower was born via surrogate to him and his wife, Grace Hightower.

I'm Not a Movie Star, but
Can I Have the Same Tests as De Niro?

Celebrities do enjoy certain perks in life, but access to testing for cancer is not one of them. Anyone with access to health—meaning nearly everyone these days—is eligible for a normal checkup, which for men of an appropriate age begins with a typical physical examination, a gathering of family medical history, and testing for prostate issues if anything suspicious is found.

What Is Prostate Cancer, and
How Is It Diagnosed?

Most men who develop prostate cancer do so because of an inherited susceptibility to the disease or as a result of damage to their DNA that occurs and accumulates during their lifetimes (more about these topics in Chapter 3).

Damage of the DNA in the cells lining the tiny glands in the prostate eventually causes these cells to "misbehave" and grow out of control—two of the hallmarks of malignancy. As the cancer progresses, these tiny glands and cells begin to look increasingly abnormal. Doctors have developed grading systems (see Chapter 1) to describe how badly these cells deviate from their normal appearance under the microscope.

A diagnosis of prostate cancer begins with a thorough family medical history. After age and race, having one or more relatives (for example, father or brothers) with prostate cancer is the most important risk factor for developing the disease. In fact, studies of twins who develop prostate cancer have shown that up to 58 percent of prostate cancer risk is related to the genes you were born with and the other 42 percent of risk is due to damage to your DNA that occurs as you age.

Your doctor will then perform a general physical examination that includes a DRE (digital rectal exam). This is when your primary care physician or urologist inserts a lubricated, gloved finger into your anus and feels the prostate gland through the wall of your rectum. The doctor checks for the size, firmness, and texture of the prostate, any hard areas, lumps, or growth spreading beyond the prostate, and any pain caused by touching or pressing on the area.

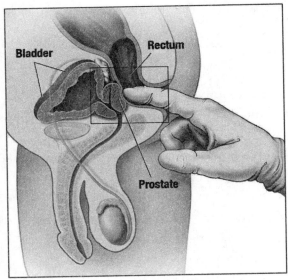

Digital Rectal Exam
Source: NCI

If you have a family history of prostate cancer/abnormalities in your DRE, your doctor will order a laboratory test to check the level of PSA in your blood and to perhaps determine how your PSA levels may have changed over time.

The University of Texas at San Antonio, Department of Urology, provides a website *(http://deb.uthscsa.edu/URORiskCalc/Pages/uroriskcalc .jsp)* where you or your doctor can plug your race, age, PSA level, family history, and DRE results into a Prostate Cancer Risk Calculator and obtain your personalized risk assessment. This assessment includes a prediction of whether or not a biopsy will be negative for cancer and the chances that you might have a low-grade or high-grade cancer (Chapter 1). You and your doctor will then discuss the pros and cons of proceeding with a biopsy of your prostate or undertaking a program of active surveillance.

A biopsy is a procedure to obtain tissue samples so a pathologist can view them under a microscope to see if cancer is present. Prostate biopsies are done through a transrectal approach. You lie on your side with your knees pulled up against your chest and your doctor inserts an ultrasound probe into your rectum to visualize your prostate gland and aim the biopsy needle. The needle is inserted ten to twelve times at different locations to pull out tiny cylinders of tissue that are placed in a preservative and sent to your pathologist.

Most cases of prostate cancer have no symptoms at first, but patients may develop or experience any of the following conditions:

- Weak or interrupted (stop-and-go) flow of urine
- Sudden urge to urinate
- Frequent urination (especially at night)
- Trouble starting the flow of urine
- Trouble emptying the bladder completely
- Pain or burning while urinating
- Blood in the urine or semen
- Pain in the back, hips, or pelvis that doesn't go away
- Difficulty in achieving an erection
- Painful ejaculation
- Shortness of breath
- Feeling very tired
- Fast heartbeat

- Dizziness
- Pale skin caused by anemia

> **NOTE to PATIENT:**
> These symptoms are not specific to prostate cancer and could also be due to other conditions, so if you have any concerns, contact your healthcare provider.

Gleason or Epstein:
I'm Confused About My Grade

A pathologist will examine your biopsy specimen under a microscope to check for cancer cells and abnormal patterns of growth. If cancer is found, the pathologist will also assign a grade (Chapter 1) to your tumor using a special grading scale.

The traditional grading system results in a Gleason score. Contrary to popular belief, the test is not named after Jackie Gleason, the legendary comedian. The name derives from a scoring system developed in 1997 by Donald Gleason, a pathologist at the Minnesota Veterans Affairs Hospital who first devised his system in the late 1960s and early 1970s.

The rise of PSA testing in the 1990s led to unintended "grade inflation" that resulted in low-grade cancers being upgraded to higher-grade (worse prognosis) tumors. In other words, a patient with a low (favorable) Gleason score would be reclassified with a higher (less favorable) Gleason score, even though the nature of his cancer hadn't really changed at all.

Statistical researchers identified this upward drift in Gleason scores as a Will Rogers phenomenon. Will Rogers (1879–1935) was an Oklahoma humorist and social commentator who once quipped, "When the Okies left Oklahoma and moved to California, they raised the average intelligence level in both states."

What this meant for prostate cancer was that because more high-grade tumors were being diagnosed while the death rates from prostate cancer remained unchanged, it appeared that cancer screening methods and modern treatment protocols were having a positive impact on prostate cancer when, in fact, they were not.

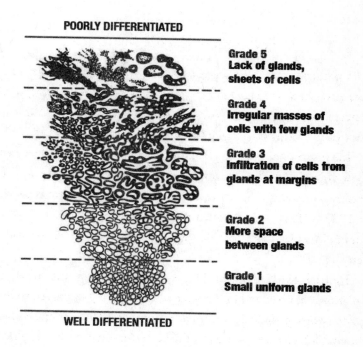

POORLY DIFFERENTIATED

Grade 5
Lack of glands,
sheets of cells

Grade 4
Irregular masses of
cells with few glands

Grade 3
Infiltration of cells from
glands at margins

Grade 2
More space
between glands

Grade 1
Small uniform glands

WELL DIFFERENTIATED

Gleason Grading
Source: Orchid Cancer Appeal (*http://www.orchid-cancer.org.uk/*)

When a pathologist receives your biopsy specimen, she or he examines your tissue under a microscope and assigns two numbers (grades) to your cancer: 1 to 5 for the predominant pattern cancer, and another 1 to 5 for the secondary pattern. So if your predominant pattern is grade 2 but your tissue contains a bit of grade 4, your Gleason score is 6 (2 + 4 = 6). Suppose the only pattern in your cancer is grade 3. This number is doubled to produce your Gleason score of 6 (3 × 2 = 6).

There are twenty five (5 × 5 = 25) combinations of numbers that can result in Gleason scores between 2 and 10. In practice, pathologists examining biopsy specimens never use grades 1 and 2, so the lowest score you'll get in your biopsy is 6.

Is that crystal clear?

No one should expect the average Joe to get this, especially the first time around, so if you are diagnosed with prostate cancer and start hearing all these numbers being tossed around, don't just sit there and let all this information mix you up. Ask your doctor to slow down and explain everything. That is their job!

The Gleason grading system underwent major revisions in 2005 and again in 2014, but it has grown even more complex and confusing for doctors and patients. Both the World Health Organization (WHO) and the International Society of Urological Pathology (ISUP) have accepted a new grading system pioneered by Dr. Jonathan Epstein, a Professor of Pathology, Oncology, and Urology at the Johns Hopkins Medical Institutions in Baltimore, Maryland. Dr. Epstein's system consists of just five grades or scores and is easier to use, easier to understand, and more accurate than the venerable Gleason system.

Here's the gist of the Epstein system.

Grade 1 tumors have no potential to metastasize, and active surveillance may be the most appropriate treatment.

Grades 2, 3, 4, and *5* have progressively less favorable prognoses and are candidates for surgical, radiation, or hormonal treatments.

For those interested in how Gleason scores compare and contrast with Epstein grades, here is a breakdown on the grading math and what it actually means regarding what a pathologist views under a microscope:

- *Epstein 1* (Gleason score of 6 or lower): only individual, discrete, well-formed glands
- *Epstein 2* (Gleason score 3 + 4 = 7): predominantly well-formed glands with a lesser component of poorly formed, fused, and/or cribriform glands
- *Epstein 3* (Gleason score 4 + 3 = 7): predominantly poorly formed, fused, and/or cribriform glands with a lesser component of well-formed glands
- *Epstein 4* (Gleason score 8): only poorly formed, fused, and/or cribriform glands, or predominantly well-formed glands with a lesser component lacking gland formation, or predominantly lacking gland formation and a lesser component of well-formed glands (but poorly formed, fused, and/or cribriform glands can be a minor component)
- *Epstein 5* (Gleason score 9–10): lacks gland formation, or has glands with necrosis with or without poorly formed, fused, and/or cribriform glands

Some doctors, such as breast cancer specialist Dr. Laura Esserman and her colleagues at the University of California School of Medicine in San Francisco, have questioned whether some low-grade conditions should even be called cancer at all. In a 2013 article in the *Journal of the American Medical Association*, Dr. Esserman and her coauthors pointed out that "the term 'cancer' often invokes the specter of an inexorably lethal condition," and that it should be reserved for conditions with a "reasonable likelihood of lethal progression if left untreated."

NOTE to PATIENT:
If you have had a biopsy and received a
Gleason score, you should request a re-grading of
your cancer by a second pathologist with experience
in the Epstein system. Do this before you and
your doctor decide on what kind of
treatment may be best for you.

MY JOURNEY

Because of a high Gleason score after my latest checkup, my urologist recommended surgery and a second opinion—but not necessarily in that order. I did my best to keep a sense of humor, had a few consults, and opted for robotic surgery. My doctor suggested that I eat well beforehand, so I filled up on tofu and vegetables and lots of organic yogurt.

My wife was thrilled—about the diet, that is. Since I'm fifty-six and she's nearly fifty, we weren't concerned that I wouldn't be a sperm-producing stud any longer, but we were kind of wondering what would happen to my "you know what." I'd heard too many depressing tales about men losing their luster, and while I certainly wanted to live, I wasn't thrilled with the notion of living the rest of my life as a male nun. I can safely say at this point, just a few months out of surgery and the immediate aftermath of recovery, that I am experiencing optimistic signs of recovering the capacity for expressing myself in the bedroom. If that continues to improve, I hope to leave cancer as a distant memory in my rearview mirror.

Fred (Providence, Rhode Island)

What Is My Stage, and How Do I Know?

Staging is a process intended to accurately assess where and how far a cancer has spread and is based on the TNM (tumor, node, and metastasis) system that we described in Chapter 1 (page 22). After your biopsy but before any further treatment, your doctor will assign a clinical stage (cTNM) based on your DRE, your biopsy interpretation and score, and either transrectal ultrasound (TRUS) or endorectal MRI imaging.

Endorectal MRI is considered to be more accurate than TRUS in detecting cancer that has grown beyond the prostate gland into neighboring tissues, such as the seminal vesicles, bladder, and rectum. TRUS is primarily used to guide your doctor in obtaining the best biopsy specimens.

Prostate cancer also spreads to lymph nodes (the N in the TNM system), starting in the pelvis and extending out from there. Distant metastases (the M of TNM) can occur when tumor cells escape into the blood stream and are carried to other tissues, most notably bone, where they land and start growing. Lymph node and bone metastases of prostate cancer are usually identified by CT scanning.

In patients with advanced disease, a special bone scan may be done if the patient is experiencing bone pain or has a PSA level greater than 20.

If your prostate is removed by surgery, a pathologic stage (pTNM) can be assigned. Examination of your prostate gland and lymph nodes by a pathologist yields a more accurate assessment of your cancer's stage than imaging studies.

- *T1* cancers cannot be felt by DRE and are not seen by imaging.
- *T2* cancers can be felt and seen but have not grown beyond the prostate gland.

- *T3* cancers have escaped beyond the prostate and grown into neighboring tissues.
- *T4* cancers have invaded the rectum, pelvis, and muscle tissues.
- *N0* cancers have not metastasized to lymph nodes, while N1 cancers have.
- *M0* cancers have not metastasized to distant sites, while M1 cancers have.

Your TNM stage is combined with other factors, such as your PSA level and Gleason score, to determine your likely prognosis.

- *Group I:* low-risk cancer, localized to the prostate (T1 or T2a) with PSA <10 and a Gleason score of 6 or less.
- *Group IIA:* localized tumor with at least one intermediate risk feature (T2b or PSA >10 or Gleason >7).
- *Group IIB:* localized tumor with at least one feature associated with a high risk for recurrence (T2c or PSA >20 or Gleason >8).
- *Group III:* cancer that has advanced beyond the prostate gland (T3).
- *Group IV:* any cancer with extensive local spread (T4) *or* lymph node metastases (N1) *or* distant metastases (M1).

MY JOURNEY

When I turned fifty, I started following my doctor's advice and had my first PSA screening. It came back a little high, but that was explained by the volume of miles I logged on my bike each week, because, as I came to find out later, when you sit on a bicycle for long stretches at a time it puts extra pressure on your perineum, which is that part between your anus and your scrotum. For some people, this can up your PSA level, even if you don't have any sign of cancer. So my doc decided I was fine. But then, about ten months later, when I did another PSA test, things started developing. My number had gone up to another level, one that didn't simply associate itself with an avid bike rider. Then after I had a digital rectal exam, my urologist said he felt something maybe a little solid, which was not a good sign, so I had a biopsy, but it was not conclusive. Over the next year my PSA numbers slowly kept rising, and another biopsy showed cancer. My doctor explained that it can be slow to develop, and that "watchful waiting" might be in order. So that's what we've been doing over the past two years. So far there has been no rush to operate or take any other drastic action. But I do get tested often, just to be safe.

Myles (Portland, Oregon)

NOTE to PATIENT:
Get a second opinion from an expert pathologist.

Active Surveillance

Imagine that you've had a needle biopsy of your prostate that revealed a Stage I, low-grade cancer. Active surveillance aims to postpone or avoid treatment until there is evidence that your cancer has progressed to a higher-risk state. Your doctor will recommend a monitoring process to periodically check for cancer progression. This process has not yet been standardized but usually involves periodic rectal exams, checking your PSA levels every three to six months, and doing a new biopsy every one to three years.

Active surveillance is safe. A 2015 Canadian study found that only 1.5 percent of nearly 1,000 men on active surveillance in 1995 died from prostate cancer twenty years later. But if they so choose and consult with their doctors, men on active surveillance can proceed with treatment any time they wish.

Ian McKellen: The Wizard Chooses a Less Aggressive Course

Sir Ian McKellen, seventy-six, most famous for playing the wizard Gandalf in *Lord of the Rings* and appearing in *The Hobbit*, told the UK's *Daily Mail*[2] that he has had prostate cancer since 2006. "When you have got it you monitor it and you have to be careful it doesn't spread. But if it is contained in the prostate it's no big deal. Many, many men die from it, but it's one of the cancers that is totally treatable so I have 'waitful watching.' I am examined regularly and it's just contained, it's not spreading. I've not had any treatment."

Sir Ian's decision to forgo surgery or radiation treatment for his prostate cancer is one option many men don't realize they may have.

According to the Prostate Cancer Foundation,[3] "Current estimates indicate that many more men are aggressively treated for prostate cancer than is necessary to save a life from the disease."

Minimally Invasive and Robot-Assisted Surgeries

How to treat your prostate cancer can be a very complicated decision because there are so many different ways to treat it and sometimes no obvious or best choice. Each treatment has pluses and minuses, and serious complications or side effects cannot always be avoided.

An operation to remove the prostate gland is called a radical prostatectomy and is performed via laparoscopic surgery, which involves

---

2. *http://www.mirror.co.uk/lifestyle/health/the-hobbits-sir-ian-mckellen-on-his-prostate-7965683*
3. *http://www.pcf.org/*

inserting tiny video cameras and surgical instruments through five small incisions in your lower abdomen. About 60 percent of laparoscopic prostatectomies in the United States are done with the assistance of a specially designed surgical robot. The best results, in terms of avoiding complications, depend on the experience of your surgeon and whether or not she or he uses a robot assistant.

Before the prostate is taken out, your surgeon will first remove a sentinel lymph node and call your pathologist to the operating room to immediately check it for cancer.

A sentinel is a guard, whose job is to keep watch. A sentinel node is the first lymph node to receive the lymphatic drainage from a tumor and the first where the cancer is likely to spread. To perform a sentinel lymph node biopsy, a blue dye is injected near the tumor. It flows through the lymph ducts to the lymph nodes. The first lymph node to receive the substance or dye is removed. A pathologist views the tissue under a microscope to look for cancer cells.

If the cancer has already escaped from your prostate, your surgeon will likely not proceed with removing your gland because the cancer has metastasized and you'll need a different kind of treatment.

If the operation proceeds, your surgeon will try to spare the nerves that run through your prostate. If they are damaged or cut, you'll probably experience complications of urinary incontinence and erectile dysfunction.

Roger Moore:
James Bond Goes Radical

Even James Bond isn't immune to prostate cancer. Sir Roger Moore, star of seven Bond movies, was diagnosed with prostate cancer in 1993 after a routine checkup and PSA testing. He underwent a radical prostatectomy one month later.

In his book *My Word Is My Bond*, Moore describes his days at home shortly after his surgery.[4] "I tumbled over and over into a well of self-pity and anger. It was the sight of my body limping its way to the bathroom with a great plastic bag attached to the other end of the garden hose that gave me the despair of inadequacy. I felt emasculated. I know I must have been completely impossible to live with."

Moore probably expressed the thoughts of many men in a similar predicament when he went on to say, "There are bits of me in specimen jars all over the world. I just hope there'll be enough of me left to put in my coffin when I die."[5]

Radiation Therapy: Beams and Seeds

Radiation to kill cancer cells can be delivered to the prostate gland externally through a beam of radiation targeted at the tumor. This is called external beam radiation, for obvious reasons. Sometimes external beam radiation goes by fancy names such as CyberKnife or Gamma Knife, which refer to particular systems that use computer-controlled robotics to target the radiation more accurately than traditional radiotherapy.

Radiation can also be delivered to the tumor by implanting 50 to 150 radioactive pellets, smaller than grains of rice, directly into the prostate gland. Treatment with these radioactive pellets or "seeds" is called brachytherapy because *brachy* in Greek means "short," and the radiation source is only a short distance from the cancer cells. Patients treated with radioactive seeds need to abstain from sex for about two weeks and then use condoms for several weeks to protect their partners from radiation exposure.

---

4. Roger Moore, *My Word Is My Bond* (New York: HarperCollins, 2009), 272.

5. *http://www.dailymail.co.uk/health/article-447671/You-live-twice—unless-youre-Roger-Moore.html #ixzz449Wq7o6A*

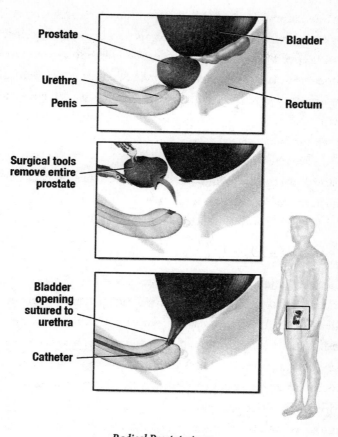

Radical Prostatectomy
Source: BruceBlaus—Own work, CC BY-SA 4.0
(https://en.wikipedia.org/wiki/Prostatectomy#/media/File:Prostate_Removal.png)

Current evidence shows that radiation therapy and surgical prostatectomy are equally effective in treating men with high-risk prostate cancer. A 2011 study reported that 92 percent of men treated with either radical prostatectomy or external beam radiation were still alive ten years later.

The two methods, however, have different side effects. A 2015 German study reported that prostatectomy patients experienced more sexual side effects and problems with urinary incontinence, while radiation therapy patients experience more bowel problems, such as diarrhea, blood in their stools, or pain in their rectums.

Hormone Therapy

Testosterone is an anabolic steroid hormone produced in the testes under the control of the pituitary gland and is responsible for male sex characteristics and normal functions of cells in the prostate gland. Testosterone is called an androgen because *andro* in Greek means "man," "male," and "masculine."

When prostate cells turn cancerous, they often still require androgen hormones to grow, so depriving prostate cancers of this androgen "fertilizer" is an important way to treat prostate cancer.

Androgen deprivation therapy can be accomplished by removing the body's natural source of testosterone—the testes—by castration, which is also known as a surgical orchiectomy. Instead of surgery, androgen deprivation can also be accomplished with drugs by using a type of chemical castration called medical orchiectomy.

Androgen deprivation therapy is a treatment option for men who are dealing with one of the following conditions:

- Cancer that has metastasized beyond the prostate gland.
- Cancer that has not escaped beyond the prostate but requires an increase in the effectiveness of external radiation therapy or a shrinking the of the prostate before brachytherapy.
- A rising PSA level after initial treatment with surgery or radiation that may signal a recurrence.

Drugs that are commonly used to lower testosterone to castration levels include leuprolide acetate (Lupron Depot) and goserelin acetate (Zoladex). These drugs are implanted under the skin as extended-release medications that can last anywhere from a month to a year.

Oral drugs that block testosterone from "fertilizing" prostate cancer cells include bicalutamide (Casodex), flutamide (Eulexin), and nilutamide (Nilandron).

Side effects of these drugs can include hot flashes, decreased libido, erectile dysfunction, breast enlargement, fatigue, weight gain, and osteoporosis. Men taking these drugs are advised to increase their dietary calcium intake and take vitamin D supplements to help protect against osteoporosis and bone fractures.

A newer drug called denosumab (Xgeva) is also available to treat bone complications of prostate cancer treatment.

Hormonal therapy may also increase the risk of heart disease.

For more information on specific drugs, we recommend the U.S. National Library of Medicine website (*http://dailymed.nlm.nih.gov/dailymed/*).

Rudy Giuliani: Combination Therapy

When the Twin Towers of the World Trade Center came down on September 11, 2001, Mayor Rudy Giuliani had to find the strength to lead a city dealing with unimaginable devastation. But as he told *Coping with Cancer*, his battle with prostate cancer, just one year earlier, had taught him some important lessons.

"It gave me a much better perspective on mortality, on life, on death, on what's really important. It gave me a great deal more empathy for what people were going through. September 11th happened close enough in time to when I went through it where I could really remember it, but long enough so that I was fully recovered, meaning

I had all of my energy back, and I was able to work for a period of time, twenty hours a day."[6]

Giuliani had been diagnosed in the spring of 2000, when a PSA test, done as part of his yearly physical examination, revealed elevated numbers. As his father had died of prostate cancer, doctors knew this result needed to be evaluated. However, when the biopsy test came back as prostate cancer, Giuliani did not rush into treatment. He thoroughly investigated all the options, taking nearly five months before making a decision.

Giuliani and his physicians put together a three-part plan. First, he would begin hormone therapy, followed by brachytherapy, followed by external beam radiation.

The hormone therapy caused hot flashes, nausea, and extreme fatigue, but he managed to continue to work through these side effects. In September 2000, he had ninety radioactive palladium pellets (each the size of a grain of rice) inserted into his prostate. Two months later, he received five weeks of five days per week external radiation therapy along with five months of adjuvant Lupron hormone therapy.

He remains cancer-free.

Targeted Focal Therapy:
Kind of Like a Lumpectomy

Instead of removing the entire prostate gland, some men can be treated with what is called focal therapy, which targets and destroys only the tumor and spares the surrounding normal tissue. Conceptually, this is like a lumpectomy for breast cancer, which surgically removes the tumor but saves the breast. However, focal therapy for prostate cancer is performed differently.

6. Laura Shipp, "A Converstation [sic] with Rudy Giuliani, Prostate Cancer Survivor," Coping with Cancer, Jan/Feb 2008, *http://copingmag.com/cwc/index.php/celebrities/celebrity_article/rudy_giuliani*

First, a special biopsy procedure is performed using a grid or template that allows your doctor to systematically sample your tissue and do a 3-D computer reconstruction, or map, of your gland. Using this map, which shows the exact location of your tumor, the surgeon places a series of temperature probes (high-tech thermometers) into your normal tissue around the tumor so that when the tumor is destroyed, the treatment doesn't go too far and damage normal tissue. The doctor then inserts freezing needles into the tumor to destroy the cancer cells.

Freezing isn't the only way to kill the cancer cells. High-intensity, focused ultrasound or lasers can also be used.

Dr. E. David Crawford is a Professor of Surgery, Urology, and Radiation Oncology at the University of Colorado and is an internationally recognized expert in the field of 3-D mapping biopsies. According to Dr. Crawford, "Targeted focal therapy is changing the landscape" of prostate cancer treatment.

Ryan O'Neal: Freezing His Future

Hollywood actor Ryan O'Neal has seen his share of cancer. The *Love Story* star was diagnosed in 2001, at the age of sixty, with chronic myelogenous leukemia (CML). Fortunately for him, it was around this time that the FDA first approved Gleevec. As O'Neal puts it, "Back then they just came out with a new miracle pill called Gleevec. It put me in complete remission. I faithfully take the pill to this day."

He spent three years at the side of his longtime love Farrah Fawcett during her ultimately unsuccessful battle with anal cancer. He was also diagnosed with skin cancer on his face, which was treated with Mohs surgery, a technique where a cancer is removed in thin layers down to normal tissue.

Then in 2014, O'Neal was diagnosed with stage T2b, Gleason 7 prostate cancer after his physician felt an abnormality during a DRE. He was referred to Dr. Duke Bahn, a diagnostic radiologist and prostate cancer specialist, where he underwent diagnostic imaging.

"After my scan, I sat down in Dr. Bahn's office and we reviewed a whole list of treatment options, including surgery, beam radiation, radioactive seeds, and targeted cryotherapy. I was particularly attracted to the cryotherapy option because of the reduced risk of side effects."[7]

O'Neal underwent the cryosurgical procedure, which Dr. Bahn calls a "male lumpectomy," and reports, "I haven't had any residual effects."

In spite of the good results O'Neal and others have experienced, Dr. Marc Garnick of Harvard Medical School recommends that because targeted cryotherapy isn't yet widely used, you should seek out a surgeon who has experience with the technique to minimize your chance of developing severe complications.

Chemotherapy for Advanced Disease

Advanced prostate cancer is sometimes called castration-resistant because it no longer responds to androgen deprivation therapy. Two chemotherapy drugs, docetaxel and cabazitaxel (Jevtana), are commonly used in this situation and are given intravenously. As with most chemotherapy drugs, patients suffer temporary but manageable side effects, including hair loss, fatigue, mouth sores, nausea, diarrhea, and low blood cell counts.

Two newer drugs, which have been described as breakthroughs in the treatment of advanced prostate cancer, are abiraterone (Zytiga) and enzalutamide (Xtandi). Abiraterone works by preventing the body from making testosterone, and enzalutamide works by replacing testosterone inside tumor cells and causing them to self-destruct.

---

7. http://pioa.org/2013/07/26/dr-bahn-ryan-oneal/

KEY POINTS TO REMEMBER

✓ If a man lives long enough, he is more likely to die *with* prostate cancer than *from* it.

✓ Routine PSA testing to detect early cancers is no longer recommended because of the risks of overdiagnosis and overtreatment.

✓ For men with low-grade tumors confined to the prostate gland, active surveillance is a safe and increasingly popular option.

✓ Men on active surveillance can change their minds and decide to undergo treatment.

✓ Surgical removal of the prostate gland is an effective treatment, but you need to understand potential complications and side effects of treatment.

✓ Radiation therapy is equally as effective as surgery and also has (different) side effects.

✓ Targeted focal therapy is kind of like a lumpectomy, but the cancer is destroyed by freezing rather than surgical removal.

✓ For cancer that has grown beyond the prostate, hormone therapy is used to starve the tumors of factors needed for growth.

✓ For patients who become resistant to hormone therapy, chemotherapy is available.

WHAT CANCER CANNOT DO

Cancer is so limited . . .
It cannot cripple love.

It cannot shatter hope.

3 CANCER, DNA, AND GENES:
It's a Family Affair

> *My cancer is me.*
> *The tumors are made of me.*
> *They're made of me as surely as my brain*
> *and my heart are made of me.*
> *It is a civil war with a predetermined winner.*
>
> —John Green, *The Fault in Our Stars*

Steve Jobs and the Cancer Genome Atlas

When Apple cofounder and former CEO Steve Jobs developed a rare type of pancreatic cancer called pancreatic neuroendocrine tumor (PNET) in 2003, he first sought answers in the realm of alternative medicine. Rather than undergo immediate surgery that might have resulted in a cure, he decided to try a vegan diet, acupuncture, herbal remedies, juice fasts, bowel cleansing, and consultation with a psychic who encouraged him to express his negative feelings. During this time, his tumor continued to grow and spread to his liver.

Eight months later, when doctors finally convinced him to have surgery, part of the tumor was analyzed for DNA mutations that might have caused or contributed to his cancer. If Jobs were lucky, the DNA analysis could reveal targets that anticancer "bullets," a new type of drug (described in Chapter 1) might attack. According to Jobs's biographer, Walter Isaacson, doctors did find some DNA mutations that led them to try targeted therapies. As a result, Jobs returned to work at Apple and continued to serve as CEO for the next three years.

In early 2009, when Jobs took a second medical leave of absence from Apple, it became clear that cancer had taken over so much of his liver that his only hope was a transplant. When doctors removed his liver, some of the cancer was analyzed again for DNA mutations, this time using more advanced technologies. Based on this testing, doctors at Stanford, Johns Hopkins, and the Broad Institute of MIT and Harvard recommended targeted drugs based on Jobs's unique set of tumor genes. He was able to return to work at Apple for about a year until his final medical leave in 2011, during which time he developed metastases to his bones. He finally passed away in October of that year, almost nine years to the date after his tumor was first detected.

When Steve Jobs had his tumor DNA analyzed in 2009, the process cost about $100,000. Today, similar testing can be done for about only $1,000. This dramatic decrease in the cost of DNA diagnostics is one important factor that has allowed government-funded, medical researchers to create The Cancer Genome Atlas (TCGA) *(http://cancer genome.nih.gov/)*. The word *genome* simply refers to every part of the DNA—the complete set of genes in our cells—that we inherited from our parents. TCGA data has vastly improved our ability to understand the genetic basis of cancer.

In fact, in May 2013, the *New York Times* declared, "Cancer will increasingly be seen as a disease defined primarily by its genetic [DNA] fingerprint rather than the organ where it originated."

But what does this mean? Can DNA be used to predict if you will get cancer? Can analysis of your DNA help you to prevent it? Can precision diagnosis using DNA lead to more effective and personalized treatments? In this chapter, we'll answer these questions by focusing on how genetics, family history, and DNA impact specific men's cancers.

Essential Facts and Definitions

Cancer is caused by mutations in the DNA that make up our genes. Human beings have about 20,000 genes, but only a few dozen are considered to be the main drivers of most tumors and are understood well enough to be useful for routine precision diagnosis and targeted treatment.

These genes come in two basic varieties:

1. *Proto-oncogenes* are normal parts of our genomes that control essential cell growth processes. Think of a proto-oncogene as the driver of a car. When chemicals or radiation in our environment permanently damage a proto-oncogene, it becomes an oncogene, and this driver not only loses control of the car, it also floors the accelerator. The most common genetic abnormality in prostate cancer is an oncogene called ERG.

2. *Tumor suppressor genes* are also normal parts of our genomes whose function is to regulate the processes of cell division and keep them in check. When tumor suppressor genes become lost or mutated, cells lose control and begin growing and dividing wildly, which is one of the hallmark behaviors of cancer. Loss or mutation of two tumor suppressor genes, PTEN and TP53, are very common in prostate cancers.

DNA mutations can occur in either germ cells or somatic cells of the body. Germ cells are either sperm or eggs and are responsible for transmitting DNA among generations from parent to child. Somatic cells are all of the other cells in your body.

DNA mutations in somatic cells (somatic mutations) are the cause of the vast majority of cancers. These cancers affect only the individual who develops them and cannot be passed on to their children. Random chance or bad luck (see Chapter 10) plays a large part in whether your DNA suffers somatic mutations that will cause you to develop cancer.

Hereditary cancers, on the other hand, are defined by permanent mutations in germ cells (or germline mutations), and the risk of developing cancer is passed between generations. Hereditary cancers are often part of familial syndromes, such as Lynch syndrome, that transmit the risk of developing several types of cancer.

Hammerin' Hank Lynch's Syndrome

Dr. Henry T. Lynch directs the Hereditary Cancer Center at the Creighton University School of Medicine in Omaha, Nebraska. In the early 1960s, while still a medical student, Lynch began gathering evidence to show that some cancers had a genetic cause. The prevailing wisdom at the time surmised that cancer was a disease caused by environmental factors, not changes in DNA, and the U.S. National Institutes of Health repeatedly turned down funding for Lynch's work. But Dr. Lynch persisted, and his research laid one of the foundations for the way we understand cancer today.

His research, and therefore his findings, almost didn't happen for reasons other than lack of funding. Before Lynch entered medical school, he was a professional boxer using the stage name "Hammerin' Hank." Perhaps this first career instilled in him the dogged determination he needed to overcome early rejection of his work by the established experts.

Lynch syndrome is a genetic condition affecting both men and women, which greatly increases their risks of developing several types of malignancies. The two most common are cancers of the colon and uterus but there may also be an increased risk of developing cancers of the stomach, small intestine, liver, pancreas, gallbladder ducts, upper urinary tract, kidney, brain and skin—and if you're male, the prostate gland. Some women with Lynch syndrome are also at increased risk of developing cancers of the ovary, and breast. Men affected by Lynch syndrome have a 50 to 80 percent chance of developing colon or rectal cancer in their lifetime, compared with only a 4.5 percent chance in unaffected individuals.

Parents who are Lynch carriers can pass this cancer susceptibility along to their children in an *autosomal dominant* pattern of inheritance. This means that there's a 50 percent chance of a child being affected if one of their parents has Lynch syndrome. Of the estimated 1 million Lynch carriers in the United States, only about five percent know they carry a mutation.

Lynch syndrome is specifically caused by defects in the machinery that fixes DNA damage in our cells and involves four DNA mismatch repair (MMR) genes, named MLH1, MSH2, MSH6 and PMS2, and a fifth gene called EPCAM. When even one of these genes is abnormal, the patient's DNA accumulates stutters that are short repetitions of the letters in their genetic code. These *stutters* are referred to as microsatellite instability or MSI, a biomarker for damage to proto-oncogenes and tumor suppressors that cause cancer.

NOTE to PATIENT:
If any type of cancer seems to run in your family, insist that your primary healthcare provider refer you to a certified genetic counselor. Or you can contact one through the National Society of Genetic Counselors at *www.nsgc.org/*.

Patients with Lynch syndrome benefit from frequent, meticulous screening procedures that are designed to catch precancerous conditions before they develop into cancer. For example, a colonoscopy is recommended every one to two years beginning between the ages of twenty and twenty-five, or every two to five years before the youngest diagnosis of colon cancer in the family—if diagnosed before the age of twenty-five. Taking aspirin or ibuprofen may be effective in reducing colon cancer risks in people with Lynch syndrome. Lowering the risk of cancer through the use of drugs or hormones is called *chemoprevention* (see Chapter 10).

The Surprising Link
Between Breast and Prostate Cancers

In 1994, after a decades-long international race, the mystery of why women in multiple generations of some families seemed doomed to develop breast and ovarian cancers was solved. Genetic research by investigators Mary-Claire King, PhD, and Mark Skolnick, PhD, isolated the first gene associated with hereditary breast cancer—the breast cancer 1 gene, or BRCA1. The National Cancer Institute of the National Institutes of Health supported this research.

Dr. James Watson, winner of the Nobel Prize for discovering the structure of DNA, said of this race, "There was no more exciting story in medical science."

Nineteen years later, in 2013, BRCA1 became famous on an entirely new level when actress and activist Angelina Jolie-Pitt announced that she had undergone surgery to remove both of her breasts and ovaries because she had inherited a defective (mutant) copy of BRCA1 from her mother and grandmother. *Without* the surgery, she had up to an 87 percent chance of developing breast cancer.

In 1995, a team of British scientists successfully cloned a second gene, BRCA2, the cause of breast cancer in certain unfortunate families. Later it was found that men who inherit abnormal BRCA2 genes have increased risks of breast, prostate, and pancreatic cancers.

Together, BRCA1 and BRCA2 launched a new era in breast and ovarian cancer prevention using the DNA of these genes to predict who was at the highest risk of developing these tumors. All of this research and discovery has led to an entirely new set of questions:

- What exactly are these BRCA genes, and how do they cause cancer?
- Should every woman be tested?
- Should men be tested?
- If the test results are abnormal, what should be done about it?

Everyone's DNA—a woman's *and* a man's—contains these two genes. So do dogs and cats, mice and rats, monkeys and all other mammals. So why don't all of these creatures get cancer?

BRCA1 and BRCA2 perform critical functions in normal cells that put the brakes on tumor formation by protecting us from environmental damage to our DNA, that is, they are tumor suppressor genes. Certain mutations deactivate or cripple these genes from performing their normal DNA repair functions. This creates a vicious cycle that leads to mutations in other oncogenes that cause and drive cancer.

In certain families, an ancestor suffered a DNA mutation in a BRCA1 or BRCA2 gene in their germ cells (eggs or sperm) and thereafter had a fifty-fifty chance of passing along the mutant gene to their sons and daughters. Such ancestors are called founders of the genetic mutation that then is passed along to many of their descendants across the generations. Descendants who inherit a defective copy of such a gene are called carriers. Medical infographics of family trees are called pedigrees.

The following pedigree provided by the National Cancer Institute, shows how BRCA2-related cancers affect three generations of a family.

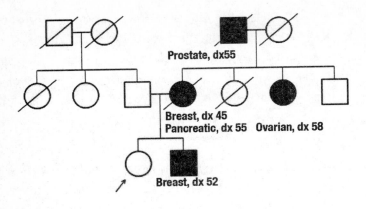

Classic BRCA2 *Pedigree*
Source: U.S. National Cancer Institute

The symbols in pedigree diagrams have special meanings. A square indicates a man, a circle stands for a woman, and a horizontal line connecting them indicates a marriage or other relationship resulting in children. If a person has a disease or other medical condition (in this case, cancer) their symbol is filled in.

The notation "dx 55" means that the person was diagnosed with cancer at age fifty-five. A long, slanted line through a square or circle indicates that the person has passed away. An arrow pointing to one of the symbols means that person is the starting point (proband) for the genetic study of the family.

> **NOTE to PATIENT:**
> Your pedigree, or detailed family medical history,
> must be part of your personal health record.

———————————————— MY JOURNEY ————————————————

I grew up in an average family in a nice suburban part of the Midwest. Bad things are not supposed to happen to us. We're supposed to live a nice life, provide for our families, try to be good neighbors, and then we're done. Or so I thought.

I was well on my way into middle age when my sister was diagnosed with breast cancer and found out she had the BRCA1 gene. Of course, I was messed up about her getting sick, but it never occurred to me that I could have this gene, too. Being a guy, it was definitely not on my radar to think about my breasts, let alone them being susceptible to getting cancer. But then my sister's oncologist recommended that I get tested, which was the smartest thing I ever did. That's because they ended up detecting breast cancer in me, and because we found it out when we did, it was treatable. And the weird thing is, I am now paying much better attention to the finer points of being alive. In fact, I would recommend it highly to anyone.

Reggie (Shaker Heights, Ohio)

Nature Versus Nurture

Are most prostate cancers inherited diseases? According to twins, the answer is yes.

Medical researchers have been studying the occurrence of cancer in more than 200,000 individual twins born since the late 1870s in the Nordic countries of Denmark, Finland, Norway, and Sweden (see *http://nortwincan.org/*). During the course of their lifetimes, some of the individuals developed cancer, and the researchers wanted to know how likely it was that their twin sibling would also develop cancer. They also wanted to know how much of any increased cancer risk was the result of nature (their genes/DNA) versus nurture (their environments).

Over the past thirty-two years, the researchers studied twenty-three different cancer types. Their latest results, published in the *Journal of the American Medical Association* in February 2016, showed that, on average, when one twin developed cancer, the co-twin had a greatly increased chance of also developing cancer. The actual lifetime risks were 46 percent for identical twins and 37 percent for fraternal twins. Identical twins share 100 percent of their DNA; whereas, fraternal twins share 50 percent (the same number of genes as ordinary siblings do), so naturally you'd expect the risk to be higher in identical twins if cancer is a disease of DNA.

The results for prostate cancer were most striking. Researchers concluded that 58 percent of the risk for developing prostate cancer is in our genes and 42 percent is due to our environments. As we pointed out in Chapter 2, your risk of developing prostate cancer is significantly higher if you have a brother or father who has been diagnosed with the disease.

> **NOTE to PATIENT:**
> Know your family history and make sure
> your doctor does, too.

John Kerry: Proving Cancer Wrong

Secretary of State John Kerry has served his country for nearly his entire adult life, beginning on the battlefields of Vietnam, then continuing as Senator from Massachusetts, then presidential candidate, and, most recently, Secretary of State. But in December 2002, when he was diagnosed with prostate cancer, Kerry realized that he needed to take some time for himself. He was already familiar with prostate cancer, having lost his father (at age eighty-five) to prostate cancer just two years earlier. "My dad had radiation, and I saw just how he lived at the end, and I didn't want to go through that," Mr. Kerry told *New York Times* reporter Lawrence Altman.[8]

After much research, Kerry decided to undergo a nerve-sparing procedure. "I was diagnosed and treated as I was crisscrossing the country running for president. So overnight, I had to put the brakes on and put my health first, halting my travel and speaking schedule. I was dead tired for weeks. But I got better, got back on the trail and picked up where I left off. I'm very proud of that. I figured I could either let this thing stop things I'd dreamed of or I could prove it wrong, and I tried my best to prove cancer wrong."[9]

PSA, DNA, and Genetic Risk Scores for Prostate Cancer

As we described in Chapter 2, PSA testing is a useful tool in the management of patients who already have prostate cancer, but it has probably caused more harm than good when used as a screening test for early detection of cancer. The harm for an individual occurs from overdiagnosis and subsequent overtreatment of a condition that may never become medically significant in that person's lifetime.

Many researchers expect that DNA testing will result in three overall improvements:

- Better selection process for men for prostate cancer screening
- Improvements in interpreting PSA levels
- Better-informed decisions about biopsies and treatment

---

8. *http://www.usrf.org/news/OCT04Kerry/kerry.htm*

9. *http://copingmag.com/cwc/index.php/celebrities/celebrity_article/john_kerry*

In addition to BRCA2 and another cancer susceptibility gene called HOXB13, about 100 other stretches of DNA are within our genomes that influence whether or not we will get prostate cancer—and how indolent or aggressive that tumor may be.

These stretches of DNA contain genetic variants called SNPs, which stands for the technical term single nucleotide polymorphisms. These SNPs are germline variations in our DNA that can be measured in a saliva sample collected by a cheek swab. Researchers are currently designing SNP-based screening tests that provide a genetic risk score for prostate cancer.

Dr. Drew Pinsky:
Get the Facts and "Don't Freak Out"

Internist, addiction specialist, and TV and radio host Dr. Drew Pinsky has made a career of helping others, so when his wife pushed him to take care of himself, Dr. Drew, as his many admirers call him, reluctantly went to his doctor, who discovered a slight but suspicious jump in the PSA level in Pinsky's blood.

"I had an extremely busy schedule and everything was catching momentum that summer," Pinsky told *patientresource.com*. "I was finally doing some things I had wanted to do. I said to myself, *Can't I at least get into all this before I get a cancer diagnosis?*"

Because his father and uncle had prostate cancer, Pinsky had been testing his PSA since he was in his mid-forties, and in 2011, at the age of fifty-three, Pinsky was diagnosed with prostatitis, an inflammation of the prostate. After two rounds of antibiotics and prostate massage, there was still no improvement, so he had a biopsy, which revealed cancer.

"My story is a good example of a physician's judgment," Dr. Drew told Jessica Webb Errickson of *Coping* magazine. "It was my internist's judgment or intuition that I should see the urologist. It was my urologist's judgment that I should be biopsied. Based on current guidelines, they would have taken a much more conservative approach."

His doctors recommended active surveillance, which meant monitoring any progression of the cancer with biopsies and PSA testing. During this time, bearing in mind his family history and the possibility of needing treatment, Dr. Drew had time to reflect on his priorities in life. "There are many options for treating early-stage prostate cancer, and you can generally take your time after diagnosis and select the best option for your particular circumstance," Dr. Drew explained in the interview. "You do not have to rush. You should not rush. Although I've had a great outcome from prostatectomy, it's intense. I really got a sense of why you'd want to pursue watchful waiting until surgery was absolutely necessary."

By the time a year of monitoring had passed, Pinsky's medical team thought surgery to remove the entire prostate was his best option. Naturally, Pinsky was concerned about losing normal functions but was relieved to discover that this was also a priority for his doctors.

It took Pinsky several months to get back to normal after his 2013 surgery, but he reported that he felt better than ever by that time and thankful that he avoided the dreaded side effects that all men worry about: erectile dysfunction and incontinence.

"I take better care of myself now," he told *PatientResource.com*. "I exercise more. I watch my diet. As a physician, you know how many bad things can happen, and I worry a little more now. But I'm paying attention and I appreciate feeling healthy."

Pinsky is still free of any cancer and dedicated to helping other men in similar situations. "I tell them, 'Don't freak out. Relax.' That's the main thing," he says. "I've laughed and cried with men who have this, and it stinks. It's not fun. You are now a member of a brotherhood you would rather not be a part of, but believe me, there are worse things."

The Critical Importance of
Genetic Counseling

If *any* kind of cancer seems to run on either side of your family, ask your primary care physician for a referral to a certified genetic counselor. Before your meeting, collect and organize your family health information and draw your own family tree. The U.S. Surgeon General's website will guide you in creating this "health portrait." *(https://familyhistory.hhs.gov/FHH/html/index.html)*

Take this information to your appointment. Because many doctors are not experts in genetics, don't be afraid to ask for a referral to a certified cancer genetic counselor. Most hospitals with cancer centers will have genetic counselors on staff. If you have trouble finding one, you can contact the National Society of Genetic Counselors *(http://nsgc .org/)* and ask for help locating a qualified counselor near you. There are also companies, such as *MyGeneCounsel.com*, that offer counseling services online or by phone. A genetic counselor will review your family medical history and recommend whether or not you should have your DNA tested.

KEY POINTS TO REMEMBER

✓ Cancer is caused by mutations in your DNA, specifically in genes that control essential biological processes (oncogenes) or genes that normally function to prevent cancer (tumor suppressor genes).

✓ Hereditary or familial cancers are caused by mutations in the DNA of germ cells (sperm or eggs) that can be passed between generations. Such mutations are called *germline mutations.*

✓ Families with Lynch syndrome have a high likelihood of developing cancers of the colon and uterus. Cancers of other regions of the gastrointestinal tract and the urinary tract (kidneys, bladder) also occur at higher rates in these families.

✓ Both of the genes that can cause breast and ovarian cancers in women, BRCA1 and BRCA2, can also lead to prostate cancer in men.

✓ Nature (your DNA) has a greater effect than nurture (your environment) on your risk of developing prostate cancer.

✓ Know your family medical history and make sure your doctor does, too.

✓ If any type of cancer seems to run in your family, seek the help of a genetic counselor to accurately assess your situation and risks.

WHAT CANCER CANNOT DO

Cancer is so limited . . .
It cannot cripple love.
It cannot shatter hope.

It cannot corrode faith.

4 TESTICULAR CANCER: A Modern Success Story in Oncology

Cancer didn't bring me to my knees.
It brought me to my feet.

—Michael Douglas

From (Almost) Certain Death to (Almost) Certain Cure

Testicular cancer is the most common cancer in men twenty to thirty-five years old. In the United States, almost 8,500 men are diagnosed with testicular cancer each year. It is also one of the most treatable, with over 95 percent of men living five years or more after their diagnoses. Fewer than 400 men die each year from the disease.[10]

Fifty years ago, 90 percent of men with advanced testicular cancer died within one year of being diagnosed. Today, more than 90 percent of these men are cured. Effective combinations of chemotherapy and refined radiation therapy—with fewer side effects—plus new surgical

---

10. *http://seer.cancer.gov/statfacts/html/testis.html*

strategies to preserve sexual function make the treatment of testicular cancer one of the biggest success stories of modern oncology.

Now the goals of treating testicular cancer have moved from simply saving a life to personalizing treatment that maximizes the patient's quality of life after being cured.

Basic Anatomy and Function

The testicles, which produce testosterone and sperm, are two egg-shaped glands located inside the scrotum (a sac of loose skin that lies directly below the penis) and are held within the scrotum by the spermatic cord, which also contains the vas deferens (the duct that carries the sperm away from the testes) and vessels and nerves of the testicles.

The testes are covered in a tough, membranous shell called the tunica albuginea. Inside them are fine-coiled tubes, called seminiferous tubules, which are lined with a layer of cells, called germ cells.

A germ cell is a type of precursor cell that ultimately gives rise to a gamete, which is a cell that fuses with another cell during fertilization, namely eggs and sperm.

Germ cells, beginning at puberty and into old age, develop into sperm cells through a number of steps, called spermatogenesis. Sertoli cells, named after Enrico Sertoli, an Italian professor at the Royal School of Veterinary Medicine in Milan in 1865, sometimes referred to as "mother" or "nurse" cells, support and nourish these developing sperm cells.

The developing sperm travel through the seminiferous tubules to the epididymis, where newly created sperm cells mature. The sperm move into the vas deferens and are eventually expelled through the urethra and out of the urethral orifice through muscular contractions.

Lying between the seminiferous tubules are cells called Leydig cells. They produce and secrete testosterone, a hormone that controls

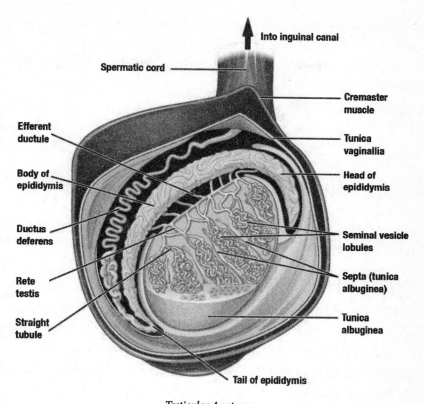

Into inguinal canal

Spermatic cord

Cremaster muscle

Efferent ductule

Tunica vaginallia

Body of epididymis

Head of epididymis

Ductus deferens

Seminal vesicle lobules

Rete testis

Septa (tunica albuginea)

Straight tubule

Tunica albuginea

Tail of epididymis

Testicular Anatomy

Source: OpenStax College—Anatomy & Physiology, Connexions Web site.
http://cnx.org/content/col11496/1.6/, Jun 19, 2013., CC BY 3.0, https://commons.wikimedia.org/w/index.php?curid=30132978

testicular volume, and other androgens—male sex hormones—which are important for sexual development and puberty, secondary sexual characteristics like facial hair, sexual behavior and libido, and supporting spermatogenesis and erectile function.

Almost all testicular cancers (95 percent) start in the germ cells. There are two main types of testicular germ cell tumors (GST): seminomas and nonseminomas, distinguished under a microscope by a pathologist. They occur in relatively even numbers but grow and spread differently and are treated differently, too. In general, nonseminomas

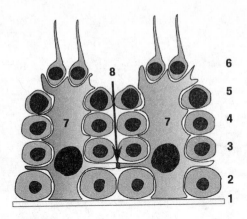

Germinal epithelium of the testicle. 1 basal lamina, 2 spermatogonia,
3 spermatocyte 1st order, 4 spermatocyte 2nd order, 5 spermatid,
6 mature spermatid, 7 Sertoli cell, 8 occlusive junctions
Source: Uwe Gille—Own work, CC BY 2.5, *https://commons.wikimedia.org/w/index.php?curid=1228766*

tend to grow and spread more quickly than seminomas. Seminomas are more likely to present with localized disease (95 percent are stage I and II) and are more sensitive to radiation. A testicular tumor that contains both seminoma and nonseminoma cells is treated as a nonseminoma.

The remaining 5 percent of testicular cancers are sex cord stromal tumors, an assortment of tumors that arise from the supporting tissues of the testes, including the Sertoli, Leydig, and granulosa cells.

_____ MY JOURNEY _____

Since I don't make it a habit to check my nut sack and my wife doesn't either, I didn't notice the swelling down there until it was too late and I had cancer. The doctor I saw was highly educated in the medical stuff, but he didn't explain much of anything, especially all these big words I had no way of knowing. When I asked him questions, he was usually too preoccupied with my charts, and when he did answer, it was like he was up on a high and mighty perch and I was down below somewhere, like a dummy. Basically, he knew what to do with my balls, but he had his head up his ass when it came to communicating with me as a human being.

Benno (Syracuse, New York)

What Are the Symptoms?

The most common symptom of testicular cancer is a painless lump or swelling in the testicle, noticed by the patient or his partner. Other symptoms include:

- A change in how the testicle feels
- A dull ache in the lower abdomen or the groin
- A sudden build-up of fluid in the scrotum
- Pain or discomfort in a testicle or in the scrotum, often described as a dull ache in the lower abdomen, the area around the anus, or in the scrotum

In about 10 percent of patients, symptoms are related to the site where the testicular cancer has already spread. For instance, a mass in the neck may signify a spread (metastasis) to the lymph nodes above the collarbones. A tumor in the lungs may cause coughing or difficulty breathing. Metastases to the skeleton can cause bone pain. Lower back pain can result from cancer spreading to the lymph nodes in the pelvis and retroperitoneum. Headaches, mental confusion, and other nervous system problems may be signs that cancer has spread to the brain.

Lance Armstrong: Shock and Awe

While this former bicyclist was revered for his athletic prowess before falling from grace in a heap of deceit and lies, his cancer experience continues to be instructive for many young men and their loved ones.

Armstrong was diagnosed with advanced testicular cancer on October 2, 1996. "I had ignored the symptoms for months; pain comes with professional cycling, so it was easy to dismiss the soreness in my groin, headaches, and difficulty breathing. I reluctantly went to the doctor after my testicle had swollen to three times its normal size. I owe a lot to my neighbor—a friend and doctor who insisted I get it checked out. By the time I was diagnosed, the cancer had already spread to my lungs and brain, so it is fair to say I was in bad shape."

Among many interviews he did over the ensuing years, which became an inspiration for many, here is what Armstrong told *MedlinePlus* magazine:

"How did I feel about it? Probably the same as anyone who has ever been diagnosed feels about cancer—I was in complete shock. Here I was, young and healthy and riding better than ever, and, suddenly, I have cancer. I was worried about losing my career and, frankly, my life. I didn't know how to tell my mom, and I was scared and angry."[11]

Now, over twenty years later, even as treatment has improved, Armstrong's cancer story continues to be instructive, as is his support of the cancer community.

Who Is at Risk for Testicular Cancer?

Anything that increases the chance of getting a disease is called a risk factor. Having a risk factor does not mean that you will get cancer, but

---

11. *https://www.nlm.nih.gov/medlineplus/magazine/issues/summer06/articles/summer06pg6-9.html*

not having risk factors doesn't mean that you will not get cancer, either. Risk factors for testicular cancer include the following:

- Having had an undescended testicle, called cryptorchidism (described in next section)
- Testicular intraepithelial neoplasia (TIN) of the testicle (described later)
- Abnormal development of the testicles
- A personal history of testicular cancer or a family history of testicular cancer, especially in a father or brother (See Chapter 3)
- Being white: the incidence of testicular cancer is four times higher in Caucasians than in African Americans

What Is Cryptorchidism?

Before a male baby is born, testicles form in his abdomen. Shortly before birth, they descend through the inguinal canal in the groin and into the scrotum.

In three out of every 100 full-term male babies, one or both testicles do not drop down like they should. In premature babies, the incidence is even higher, with up to 30 out of 100 having undescended testicles. The undescended testicles may be lying up in the lower abdomen or in the groin area.

For 70 percent of babies, the undescended testicles will drop into the correct position by the time the baby is six months old. Although these testicles can be healthy and normal, sometimes they do not develop correctly or function as they should. A testicle that does not fully descend can become damaged and, ultimately, leads to infertility or other medical problems.

The goal of treatment for undescended testicles is to bring them down into the correct place in the scrotum. Most doctors believe that the best time to do this is while the child is still young—between six and eighteen months of age.

Men who have had undescended testicles (one or both, whether treated or not) may have an increased risk for testicular cancer. It is important for men and teenage boys who have had this condition to examine their testicles each month to feel for lumps or other signs of tumors or problems.

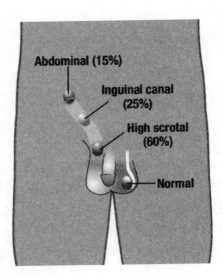

Undescended Testicle

MY JOURNEY

I don't care what you're made of or how macho you think you are. When it comes to getting cancer, everybody needs help. Everybody. Big dudes, tough guys, jocks, gang members—it don't matter. Cancer will mess you up and bring you to your knees. And if you think you can handle it all by yourself, you're an idiot. Who doesn't need support, at least some kinda help, when their normal life gets hijacked, almost overnight? And it don't matter who helps you, or how. Take what you can get, say thank you, and then try to help somebody else who's suffering like you. Believe me, we all need it.

Bobby (Elmira, New York)

How Is Testicular Cancer Diagnosed?

Six methods are available for detecting and diagnosing testicular cancer.

1. *Physical examination and history.* Your examination will begin with a complete medical history, including your health habits, past illnesses, and treatments. Your family history is also important. Your healthcare provider will perform a head-to-toe physical examination. Then, the physician will examine your testicles, checking for lumps, swelling, or pain.

2. *Ultrasound exam* uses high-energy sound waves (ultrasound) that are bounced off internal tissues or organs and make echoes, which form a picture of body tissues, called a sonogram. Ultrasound used in the detection of testicular cancer is very accurate and can detect a tumor as small as one to two millimeters in diameter.

   Seminomas and nonseminomas look somewhat different on a sonogram. Seminomas tend to be well-defined and don't have any cystic areas (seen as dark spaces in these images). On the other hand, nonseminomas look heterogeneous, with areas of calcifications (seen as white specks), cystic areas, and indistinct edges.

   Although detecting tumors works well with ultrasound, staging a tumor (see Chapter 1) with ultrasound is inaccurate.

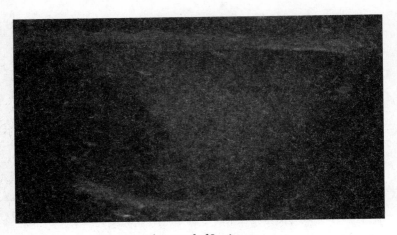

Ultrasound of Seminoma

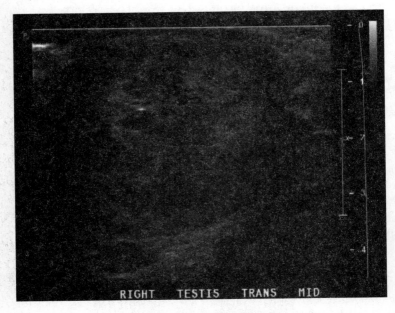

Ultrasound of Non-Seminoma

Source: Dr Laughlin Dawes (through Creative Commons)

The main reason is that the tunica albuginea, which surrounds the testis, is difficult to see on ultrasound; therefore, it is hard to tell whether the tumor is confined to the testicle or not.

3. **Serum tumor markers.** A sample of blood is examined to measure the amounts of certain substances released into the blood by organs, tissues, or tumor cells in the body. Certain substances can be linked to specific types of cancer when found in increased levels in the blood. These are called tumor markers.

   Testicular cancer has three serum tumor markers: alpha-fetoprotein (AFP), beta-human chorionic gonadotropin (β-hCG), and lactate dehydrogenase (LDH).

   Eighty to 85 percent of men diagnosed with nonseminomas have elevated levels of AFP/β-hCG, even when their disease is confined to the testicle. In contrast, less than 20 percent of men with seminoma have an elevated β-hCG while the AFP level is not elevated. Although elevated β-hCG/AFP is suggestive of testicular cancer, the diagnosis is not considered confirmed until a pathologist examines testicular tissue and verifies the finding.

4. **Radical inguinal orchiectomy** removes the entire testicle through an incision made in the groin. A tissue sample from the testicle is then viewed under a microscope to check for cancer cells.

   Unlike surgeries to diagnose cancer in other organs, in the case of testicular cancer, the surgeon does not cut through the scrotum into the testicle to remove a sample of tissue for biopsy. The reason is that if cancer is present, the procedure could cause it to spread into the scrotum and lymph nodes. It's important to choose a surgeon who has experience with this kind of surgery. If cancer is found, the cell type (seminoma or nonseminoma) is determined in order to help plan treatment.

As the testicle with cancer has been removed in its entirety during this procedure, it is considered both diagnostic and therapeutic.

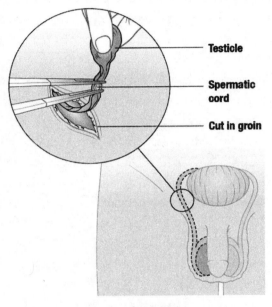

Testicle

Spermatic cord

Cut in groin

Inguinal Orchiectomy
Source: Cancer Research UK—Original email from CRUK, CC BY-SA 4.0,
https://commons.wikimedia.org/w/index.php?curid=34333438

NOTE to PATIENT:
Any man undergoing an inguinal orchiectomy
should be informed of fertility preservation methods
prior to the procedure. Semen cryopreservation should
be made available prior to instituting therapy.
This is discussed in detail in Chapter 9.

5. ***Computed tomography*** (CT) images of the abdomen and pelvis are useful in determining the extent of tumor spread. Enlarged lymph nodes in the retroperitoneum (lower abdomen and pelvis) are readily seen on a CT scan or MRI. However, there is a high rate of false negative (as high as 45 percent) because CT scan images cannot detect microscopic cancer cells (micrometastases) present in a significant number of men with testicular cancer.

6. ***Retroperitoneal lymph node dissection*** (RPLND) is a surgical procedure in which lymph nodes in the abdomen are removed and a sample of tissue is checked for signs of cancer.

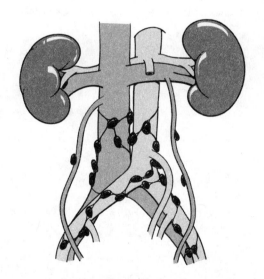

Retroperitoneal Lymph Nodes
Source: ©2016, Memorial Sloan Kettering Cancer Center (with permission)

In addition to helping to establish its exact stage and type, RPLND is also used to treat testicular cancer. It is usually performed using an incision that extends from the sternum (breastbone) to several inches below the navel. But not all men are candidates for RPLND.

— MY JOURNEY —

When my dad got skin cancer years ago, he wouldn't talk about it at all, like he had brought a big fat sin into the house that he had to pretend wasn't there. He was so ashamed to have cancer that I thought I would come home one day and find an exorcist trying to rid him of it, as if that was even possible. So when I got testicular cancer recently, I didn't have to think too hard about whether I could tell anyone. It was a no-brainer. Having the cancer is hard enough, and this kind is particularly embarrassing in some ways, but keeping it all hush-hush is downright idiotic. I hope that in this day and age, men who get this will feel okay to talk about it, because it helps a lot to let it out and get some support from people in your life. I don't talk much with my dad about it, because it just reminds him of his own past, and, besides, I don't need him telling me lousy jokes about what I should be doing with my own body.

Kevin (Chapel Hill, North Carolina)

Staging Testicular Cancer

Testicular cancer spreads in a well-known pattern, and the lymph nodes in the retroperitoneum are a primary landing site during spread of the disease. Examining the removed lymphatic tissue will determine the extent of spread of any malignant disease, and if no malignant tissue is found, the cancer may be more accurately considered stage I cancer, that is, limited to the testis.

The process used to discover if cancer has spread within the testicles or to other parts of the body is called staging, which we introduced in Chapter 1. The information gathered from the staging process determines the stage of the disease. It is important to know the stage in order to plan treatment. Some of the tests used to stage testicular cancer include the following:

- *Chest X-ray* is an X-ray of the organs and bones inside the chest.
- *CT scan* is a procedure in which a computer linked to an X-ray machine makes a series of detailed pictures of areas inside the body and taken from different angles. A dye may be swallowed or injected into a vein to help the organs or tissues show up more clearly.
- *Abdominal lymph node dissection* surgically removes lymph nodes in the abdomen, and a sample of tissue is checked for signs of cancer. This procedure is also called a lymphadenectomy. For patients with nonseminoma, removing the lymph nodes may help stop the spread of disease. Cancer cells in the lymph nodes of seminoma patients can be treated with radiation therapy.
- *Serum tumor marker test*, as mentioned earlier, measures serum tumor markers during the diagnosis phase of cancer. They are measured again after an inguinal orchiectomy and a biopsy to determine the stage of the cancer. This helps to show if all of the cancer has been removed or if more treatment is needed. Tumor marker levels are also measured during follow-up as a way of checking if the cancer has come back.

For men with disseminated seminomas, the main adverse prognostic variable is the presence of metastases in organs other than the lungs (e.g., bone, liver, or brain). For men with disseminated nonseminomas, the following variables are associated with a poor prognosis:

- Metastases to organs other than the lungs
- Highly elevated serum tumor markers
- Tumor that originated in the mediastinum rather than the testis

Nonetheless, even patients with widespread metastases at the time of diagnosis, including those with brain metastases, may have curable disease and should be treated with this intent.

Stages of Testicular Cancer

Stage	Examples	Tumor Markers
Stage 1A	The tumor is in the testicle and epididymis and may have spread to the inner layer of the membrane surrounding the testicle.	All are normal.
Stage 1B	The tumor is in the testicle and the epididymis and has spread to the blood vessels or lymph vessels or the outer layer of the membrane surrounding the testicle, the spermatic cord or the scrotum.	All are normal.
Stage 1S	Cancer is found anywhere within the testicle, spermatic cord, or the scrotum.	All tumor marker levels are slightly above normal; or one or more tumor marker levels are moderately above normal or high.
Stage IIA	Cancer is anywhere within the testicle, spermatic cord, or scrotum and has spread to up to 5 lymph nodes in the abdomen. None are larger than 2 cm.	All tumor marker levels are normal or slightly above normal.
Stage IIB	Cancer is anywhere within the testicle, spermatic cord, or scrotum and either: • has spread to up to 5 lymph nodes in the abdomen; at least one of the lymph nodes is larger than 2 centimeters, but none are larger than 5 centimeters; or • has spread to more than 5 lymph nodes; the lymph nodes are not larger than 5 centimeters.	All tumor marker levels are normal or slightly above normal.

Stage IIC	Cancer is anywhere within the testicle, spermatic cord or scrotum and has spread to a lymph node in the abdomen that is larger than 5 centimeters.	All tumor marker levels are normal or slightly above normal.
Stage IIIA	Cancer is anywhere within the testicle, spermatic cord, or scrotum and may have spread to one or more lymph nodes in the abdomen and has spread to distant lymph nodes or to the lungs.	All tumor marker levels are normal or slightly above normal.
Stage IIIB	Cancer is anywhere within the testicle, spermatic cord, or scrotum and may have spread to one or more lymph nodes in the abdomen, to distant lymph nodes or to the lungs.	The level of one or more tumor markers is moderately above normal
Stage IIIC	Cancer is anywhere within the testicle, spermatic cord, or scrotum and may have spread to one or more lymph nodes in the abdomen, to distant lymph nodes or to the lungs.	The level of one or more tumor markers is high.
OR	Cancer is anywhere within the testicle, spermatic cord, or scrotum and may have spread to one or more lymph nodes in the abdomen, and has not spread to distant lymph nodes or the lung but has spread to other parts of the body.	Tumor marker levels range from normal to high.

Source: Celebrity Diagnosis

Testicular Intraepithelial Neoplasia (TIN)

This is sometimes considered to be stage 0, when abnormal cells are found in the tiny tubules where the sperm cells begin to develop. These abnormal cells are generally regarded as a precursor to germ cell testicular cancers. TIN is considered noninvasive and is confined to the seminiferous tubules. All tumor marker levels are normal.

TIN is often found in the tissue adjacent to germ cell cancers. It is also found in men at higher risk for testicular cancer, such as those with cryptorchidism, testicular cancer in the other testis, as well as other abnormalities of gonad development. It is sometimes found in men who are involved in an infertility evaluation and undergo a testicular biopsy.

TIN may or may not progress to invasive germ cell tumors, either seminomas or nonseminomas. The actual risk of progression and the latency period is currently unknown; therefore, the management of TIN remains controversial, especially in men with TIN on one side only. Options include observation, surgical removal of the testis, and low-dose radiation therapy.

Jake Gibb: From Beach Ball to Blood Tests

If you are a professional beach volleyball fan, you may remember Jake Gibb, who represented the United States as a player in the 2008 Beijing Olympics.

In 2010, while training to make the team for the 2012 London Games, Jake received a call from the U.S. Anti-Doping Agency, which informed him that he had failed a routine drug test because he had tested positive for β-hCG and AFP.

"I was just absolutely thrown," Jake says in an interview with *Coping with Cancer*[12] magazine. He looked up the two drugs and found out that they were mostly found in pregnant women and in steroid abusers. Jake was neither!

"At the very bottom of this article, there was one line that said, 'Also found in men with testicular cancer,'" he explained, "and my heart just dropped."

---

12. *http://copingmag.com/cwc/index.php/celebrities/celebrity_article/jake_gibb*

Jake's diagnosis was confirmed. He was originally told that he would have to undergo three rounds of chemotherapy after surgical removal of the cancer. This would have eliminated any chance for him to train and, hopefully, qualify for the Olympic team.

After his surgery, Gibb found out that chemo or radiation therapy would not be necessary. This was what Gibb called, "The biggest relief . . . and joy of my life!"

Gibb, along with his partner, Sean Rosenthal, went on to represent the United States in beach volleyball at the 2012 Olympics, finishing in fifth place; however, that same year, he and Rosenthal finished first in world on the FIVB (Fédération Internationale de Volleyball) tour.

Treatment Options

As with many cancers, certain factors affect prognosis (chance of recovery) and choices for treatment. For testicular cancer, they include the following:

- Stage of the cancer (whether it is in or near the testicle or has spread to other places in the body, and blood levels of AFP, β-hCG, and LDH)
- Size of the tumor
- Number and size of retroperitoneal lymph nodes

Testicular cancer is highly treatable and usually curable. For treatment planning, germ cell tumors are broadly divided into seminomas and nonseminomas because they have different prognostic and treatment algorithms. For patients with seminoma (all stages combined), the cure rate exceeds 90 percent. For patients with low-stage seminoma or nonseminoma, the cure rate approaches 100 percent.

For most men, treatment begins with surgery—a radical inguinal orchiectomy, done at the time of diagnosis. The primary exception to this is a patient with a life-threatening, advanced disease. They will undergo chemotherapy prior to orchiectomy. Recommendations for further treatment after orchiectomy depend upon the stage of the cancer as well as the tumor's histology, that is, what a pathologist sees under the microscope.

Testicular tumors are divided into three groups, based on how well they are expected to respond to treatment.

1. Good Prognosis

For nonseminoma, all of the following must be true:

- The tumor is found only in the testicle or in the retroperitoneum (area outside or behind the abdominal wall).
- The tumor has not spread to organs other than the lungs.
- The levels of all the tumor markers are slightly above normal.

For seminoma, all of the following must be true:

- The tumor has not spread to organs other than the lungs.
- The level of alpha-fetoprotein (AFP) is normal. Beta-human chorionic gonadotropin (β-hCG) and lactate dehydrogenase (LDH) may be at any level.

2. Intermediate Prognosis

For nonseminoma, all of the following must be true:

- The tumor is found in one testicle only or in the retroperitoneum (area outside or behind the abdominal wall).
- The tumor has not spread to organs other than the lungs.
- The level of any one of the tumor markers is more than slightly above normal.

For seminoma, all of the following must be true:

- The tumor has spread to organs other than the lungs.
- The level of AFP is normal. β-hCG and LDH may be at any level.

3. Poor Prognosis

For nonseminoma, at least one of the following must be true:

- The tumor is in the center of the chest between the lungs.
- The tumor has spread to organs other than the lungs.
- The level of any one of the tumor markers is high.

There is no poor prognosis grouping for seminoma testicular tumors.

For most men with stage I disease, orchiectomy is curative; however, over 95 percent of recurrences occur within the first two years after orchiectomy, and half of these occur in the retroperitoneal lymph nodes. CT scans (or MRIs) can visualize these enlarged lymph nodes; however, they cannot detect microscopic amounts of tumor cells.

Some men decide to have a retroperitoneal lymph node dissection. The procedure can detect these micrometastases. But 70 percent of men who undergo RPLND have no detectable tumor and do not benefit from the surgery.

Other men, in lieu of RPLND, will choose to undergo chemotherapy, radiation therapy, or a strict active surveillance program.

An in-depth discussion of your treatment options with your healthcare team will help you make the appropriate decision to meet your specific needs.

--------------------- MY JOURNEY ---------------------

I don't know which was worse: keeping an eye on it for months and months and months, with tests and blood counts all the time, worrying about whether it would stay cool or get worse; or the treatment I finally had, and the side effects. It's a toss-up, I guess, and each man has to make his own decision how to approach it. For me, it really helped to talk with my doctor, and I was lucky that he listened to my concerns and answered all my questions, whether that was in person or through emailing back and forth. I really thank him for that.

Cedric (Houston, Texas)

Active Surveillance

Men who have stage I cancer without any additional high-risk factors may opt for active surveillance. As was the case for Sir Ian McKellen's prostate cancer (Chapter 2), active surveillance is not just waiting around to see if the cancer returns. Specific protocols are to be followed, including blood work and radiologic examinations. They are summarized here:

Protocol for Active Surveillance			
	Physical Exam and Serum Tumor Markers (AFP, hCG, LDH)	CT Scan	Chest X-Ray
Seminoma			
Year 1	Every 3–6 months	At 3, 6, and 12 month	Only if indicated clinically
Years 2 and 3	Every 6–12 months	Every 6–12 months	
Year 4 and beyond	Each year	Every 1–2 years	
Nonseminoma			
Year 1	Every 2 months	Every 4-6 months	Type IA : Months 4 and 12

			Type I B: Every 2 months
Year 2	Every 3 months	Every 4-9 months	Type IA: Every year
Years 3 and 4	Every 4-6 months	Every year	Type 1B:
Year 5 and beyond	Every year	Every year	Gradually decreased to every year by Year 5

Source: Celebrity Diagnosis

Radiation Therapy

Radiation therapy is a cancer treatment that uses high-energy X-rays or other types of radiation to kill cancer cells. It is primarily used as an adjunctive (additional) therapy for men who have undergone orchiectomy. It is used primarily for patients with seminoma, because this type of tumor is sensitive to radiation and can be used in low doses. Radiation therapy can prevent relapse in 96 percent or more of patients with stage I seminoma.

During radiation therapy, you will be lying faceup on a table. A shield is placed around the remaining testis to decrease the amount of radiation exposure to it. The radiation field is in the shape of a hockey stick, which covers both the lymph nodes in the groin of the affected side, as well as on both sides of the aorta in the pelvis and abdomen.

Chemotherapy

Men with stage I seminoma who do not wish to do active surveillance, or who want more aggressive treatment (even though their prognosis is good), may be given one or two rounds of a chemotherapy agent called carboplatin.

For men with stage I nonseminoma, as well as men with stage II and III seminomas and nonseminomas, chemotherapy in the form of bleomycin, etoposide, and cisplatin (BEP) is frequently recommended. The number of rounds of chemotherapy is based on the extent of the disease. This combination is also used for advanced and recurrent disease.

Scott Hamilton: Badge of Honor

After his gold medal victory in figure skating at the 1984 Olympics, Scott Hamilton was riding high in his athletic career. In 1997, while touring with *Discover Stars on Ice*, he began experiencing pain in his abdomen. "I knew something was going on," he said, "but I didn't know what. I thought it was an ulcer or stress or lifestyle. By the time I got a checkup from a doctor, I had a tumor in my abdomen that was twice the size of a grapefruit. That should never happen—ever! I'm so in touch with my body that for me to let it get to that point was stupid."[13]

That tumor turned out to be testicular cancer. After his orchiectomy, Scott underwent twelve weeks of chemotherapy with bleomycin and etoposide. "I had my bleomycin every Friday," he told *Menweb. org.*[14] "I hated bleo Fridays. That particular drug affects your lungs and I still feel my stamina isn't what it was. But it is getting better. A lot of the other chemo affects your skin, and I have streaks of tan skin and that reminds me of everything. I also have a scar—but it's like a badge of honor. There is always going to be something, some challenge. It's important not to shy away from it."

Hamilton went on to skate again, including Ice Capades and *Scott Hamilton's Celebration on Ice*. He also worked on TV as a figure skating commentator and became an inductee into the halls of fame for

---

13. *http://copingmag.com/cwc/index.php/celebrities/celebrity_article/scott_hamilton*
14. *http://www.menweb.org/tcscotth.htm*

the U.S. Olympics and the World Figure Skating Championships. In 1999, he started the Scott Hamilton CARES Initiative, with an emphasis on funding cancer research, sharing online information on chemotherapy and providing one-on-one mentorship for patients.

Which Treatment Is Right for Me?

The following two algorithms outline the decision tree for treating men with testicular cancer.

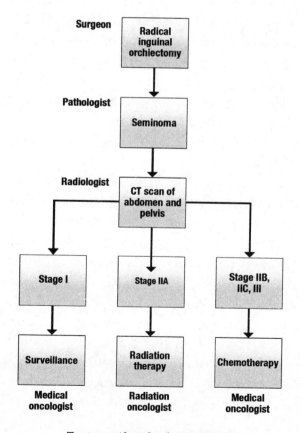

Treatment Algorithm for Seminomas
Source: Celebrity Diagnosis

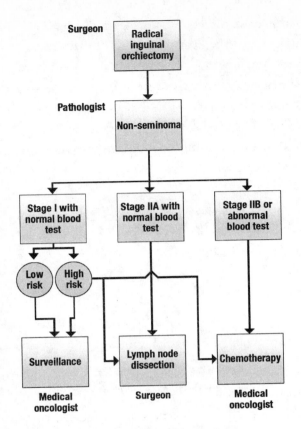

Treatment Algorithm for Non-Seminomas
Source: Celebrity Diagnosis

Possible Side Effects of Treatment

The National Cancer Institute reports that out of 100 patients receiving BEP, fewer than twenty and up to 100 may experience the following side effects, some of which are common, while others may be serious:

- Skin changes
- Peeling skin

- Changes in skin color
- Hair loss
- Fever
- Mouth sores, which may cause difficulty swallowing
- Scarring of the lungs, which may cause shortness of breath
- Diarrhea, loss of appetite, nausea, vomiting
- Infection, especially when white blood count is low
- Anemia, which may require blood transfusions
- Bruising, bleeding
- Kidney damage, which may cause swelling and may require dialysis
- Hearing loss, including ringing in the ears
- Chills
- Fatigue

Out of 100 patients receiving BEP, from four to twenty may experience these occasional side effects, some of which may be serious:

- Blood clot, which may cause swelling, pain, and shortness of breath
- Heart failure or heart attack, which may cause chest pain, shortness of breath, swelling of ankles, and fatigue
- Stroke, which may cause paralysis, weakness, headache
- Sores on the skin
- Liver damage, which may cause yellowing of eyes and skin, and swelling
- Confusion
- Swelling of the brain
- Blood in urine
- Allergic reaction, which may cause rash, low blood pressure, wheezing, shortness of breath, swelling of the face or throat and possibly even death

- Difficulty with balance
- Severe skin rash with blisters and peeling, which can involve the lining of the mouth and other parts of the body

Out of 100 patients receiving BEP, three or fewer may experience rare, albeit serious, side effects, such as cancer of the bone marrow (leukemia, which is caused by having chemotherapy later in life) or seizures.

> **NOTE to PATIENT:**
> For more information about side effects from testicular cancer treatment, see Chapters 7 and 8.

KEY POINTS TO REMEMBER

✓ Cancer of the testicle is most common in younger men, ages fifteen to thirty-five.

✓ The most important risk factor for developing testicular cancer is an (untreated) undescended testicle.

✓ The second most important risk factor is having a close relative, such as a brother, with the disease.

✓ The two main types of testicular cancer are seminoma and nonseminoma.

✓ Blood tests are often useful for diagnosis, staging, and monitoring response to therapy.

✓ Greater than 90 percent of men diagnosed with cancer of the testicles can be cured.

✓ Some patients may suffer long-term consequences of chemotherapy and radiation therapy.

✓ There are ways to preserve fertility and reproductive functions after treatment.

WHAT CANCER CANNOT DO

Cancer is so limited . . .
It cannot cripple love.
It cannot shatter hope.
It cannot corrode faith.

It cannot eat away peace.

5 STRANGE BUT TRUE: Breast Cancer in Men

Don't sit around playing Mr. Tough Guy.
Don't say, "It's going to go away."
It's important, just go get checked out.
It's not like you're going to lose your manhood.

—Peter Criss, former Kiss drummer, as told to *rollingstone.com*

Yes, It Can Happen to You

If you surveyed most any random group of average American citizens and asked them about the chance of men getting breast cancer, most of them would probably shrug their shoulders, surprised at the question, and answer somewhere in the range of slim to none—and they would be right.

According to the National Institute of Health's National Cancer Institute, less than one percent of all breast cancers occur in men. A man's lifetime risk of being diagnosed with breast cancer is about one in 1,000. In contrast, a women's lifetime risk of developing breast cancer is one in eight.

But it can happen, and it does. As Peter Criss once said, "You don't need boobs to get breast cancer."

Because breast cancer in men is so rare, projected to affect approximately 2,600 men in 2016, it has been difficult for scientists to study it, and most of the rationale for treating it derives from research and experience with female breast cancer.

Most of the time this strategy works because breast cancers in men and women are more alike than different; however, breast cancer usually occurs at an older age in men than in women, and the tumors are larger and usually present at a more advanced stage.

Basic Anatomy and Function

The anatomy of a man's breast is similar in many ways to that of a woman's. Both arise from the same fetal tissues. They develop in an identical manner until the individual reaches puberty. At that time, under the influence of estrogens, breast tissue enlarges and develops. Males produce very little estrogen. Instead, they make testosterone and other androgens, that is, hormones that stimulate or control the development and maintenance of male characteristics. As a result, breast tissue in men does not develop to the same extent as it does in females. Lobules, the glands that produce milk in the female breast, do not form in the male breast.

The male breast is located between the pectoral muscles and the subcutaneous tissues, which are the tissues under the skin. Like the female breast, it is made up mostly of a fatty tissue, called adipose tissue. In addition to fat cells, the breast contains a network of ligaments and fibrous connective tissue that helps support it. The breast also features nerves that provide various sensations; blood and lymphatic vessels to bring oxygen, nutrients, and infection-fighting cells; lymph nodes and lymphatic channels that drain and filter body fluids and cells.

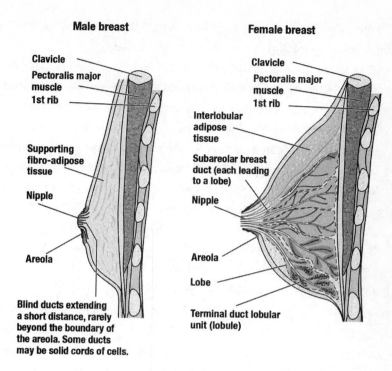

Comparison of the Male to Female Breast
Source: Peter Lamb (through *123rf.com*)

MY JOURNEY

I had heard plenty of stories about women discovering lumps in their breasts while showering and then finding out they have breast cancer. Even when I felt something in my chest, it never occurred to me that I could have cancer. At first, I figured it was a pimple or something, those annoying ones that grow under the skin and can stay there for a long time—and they hurt! It lingered for a long time, so then I thought it must be a cyst or something like that but definitely not cancer, not breast cancer, that's for sure. As far as I knew, men didn't get that. The men I know don't even refer to that part of their body as a breast. It's your chest, for crying out loud. I mean, I had never heard of men having breast cancer—ever—and I consider myself decently intelligent and fairly well read.

So after about a year had passed, I decided to go for a physical, because after turning sixty I was due for another colonoscopy, too. I almost forgot to mention the thing in my chest until my doctor accidently bumped his stethoscope into me and I reacted, 'cause it hurt. He prodded and poked a little and then he got this look on his face like he was worried, so I said, "What?"

One thing led to another and I became a lousy statistic, one of those very unlucky men—there are not many, I found out—who have breast cancer. And I was *really* unlucky, because I waited so long to get checked out and the cancer had actually spread by then, so now I'm not doing so good, and I have no one but myself to blame for that.

Phillip (Atlanta, Georgia)

Risk Factors

Most men with breast cancer had no identifiable risk factors. For example, Hispanic and Asian men have the lowest risk of developing breast cancer. Caucasian men have double the risk, and African American men have about two-and-a-half times the risk compared with Hispanic and Asian men.

But a number of factors are associated with its development. Certain genetic conditions, such as Klinefelter syndrome, or being a carrier of hereditary breast cancer genes, BRCA1 and BRCA2 (Chapter 3), increase the risk. Liver diseases, such as cirrhosis, that raise estrogen levels in men increase the risk of developing breast cancer.

Other factors that may increase a man's risk include radiation to the chest, lifestyle habits—such as obesity and alcohol abuse—and workplace exposures, for example, high temperatures/exhaust fumes.

Men may develop breast cancer at any age, but it is usually detected in men sixty to seventy years old. Patients younger than this may be carriers of hereditary breast cancer genes.

Richard Roundtree:
Giving Voice to a Silent Minority

Since his portrayal of private detective John Shaft in the iconic 1970s film franchise *Shaft*, actor Richard Roundtree is known as "the first black action hero" and the personification of masculinity. So imagine his disbelief when he was diagnosed with breast cancer in 1993.

He underwent a modified radical mastectomy, followed by six months of intensive chemotherapy. He talked about his diagnosis years later in a 2009 *Essence* interview:

"I'm blessed because I'm somewhat of a hypochondriac, and while I was taking a shower in Costa Rica I felt this lump. I knew it wasn't ordinary, so I finished work about a week later and had my doctor check it out. He said it's nothing to worry about but let me stick a needle in it anyway. Three days later I received the we-need-to-talk call that immediately sent up red flags for me like crazy. When he sat me down and told me I had cancer so many things went through my mind but the first was, "Wait, did he just say I had breast cancer?" That word scared the beejeezus out of me! I couldn't relate and I thought he was questioning my manhood because women die from this, not men. How could I possibly have that? But I soon learned that this disease is not gender-based."[15]

---

15. *http://www.essence.com/2009/10/10/richard-roundtree-on-surviving-breast-ca*

For several years after his diagnosis, Roundtree hid his illness, afraid he could lose his acting career. It wasn't until he was cancer-free for five years, while at an annual celebrity golf benefit for breast cancer screening, that he blurted out, "I'm so happy to hear that free screenings are being made available because I'm a breast cancer survivor!"[16]

Although his statement was initially met with shock, a tremendous outpouring of support quickly followed. He immediately became a symbol for the previously silent minority of men who get the disease.

Signs and Symptoms

Most men get diagnosed with breast cancer because they discovered a hard, painless lump in the breast. You might think that detecting a lump in a man would be easy, because the average size of a tumor at the time of diagnosis is larger in men than in women. But because of a lower general awareness among men—and their tendency to deny and delay—they are less likely to believe that a lump can actually be dangerous, let alone a sign of breast cancer. As a result, they often delay seeking medical advice.

Not all breast lumps in men are cancer, either. They can be caused by a variety of other conditions, such as infections or gynecomastia, which is an enlargement of the male breast because of a hormonal imbalance.

A tissue biopsy will often be needed for a definitive diagnosis. If it shows cancer, the patient will undergo a TNM staging work-up, as described in Chapter 1, before surgery is performed or other treatments are started.

---

16. *http://copingmag.com/cwc/index.php/celebrities/celebrity_article/richard_roundtree*

Peter Criss: Early Detection Saved My Life

George Peter John Criscuola—better known as Peter Criss—became rock music royalty as the drummer and one of the original members of the band Kiss. He was best known for his "Catman" persona, stating on more than one occasion that he felt he must have had nine lives to survive his rough upbringing on the streets of Brooklyn, New York.

After a normal workout at the gym in 2007, Criss noticed a painful lump in his left breast.

"As a man, I thought I must have pulled a muscle, and being in spandex and lipstick and high heels most of my life, I'm pretty used to my body. I just felt like something was wrong and I told my wife so she mentioned it to the doctor. He said if you were my husband I would send you over to New York Presbyterian to see Dr. Switzel.

"But that's a cancer hospital for women. She goes, 'Yeah, but I think you should go there.' It blew my mind walking into a huge room like this with nothing but women, no men, except for their husbands with them. It felt really uncomfortable for me, and it actually scared the pants off of me."

Criss underwent a lumpectomy to remove what was initially thought to be a harmless nodule. But the mass turned out to be breast cancer and he underwent a mastectomy. Fortunately, because the cancer was caught early, Criss did not need chemotherapy, and has remained cancer free.

Criss says he learned that breast cancer ran in his family, so he called his sisters, nieces, daughter, and even his brother about possible risks. Since then, he has become an outspoken advocate for breast cancer—especially when it comes to raising awareness in men.

"Every year, I meet twenty eighteen-year-old boys (who have breast cancer) and they don't know what to do. They're embarrassed. It's a chick's disease. Only girls get it.

"My battle is I just want guys to know they can get it, and if they can detect it immediately [they can be cured]. [Early detection] saved my life and I've now become very involved."[17]

What Kinds of Breast Cancer Do Men Get, and Why Does It Matter?

For the most part, men get the same kinds of breast cancer as women. Infiltrating ductal carcinoma is cancer that has spread beyond the cells that line ducts in the breast. This is the most common type, representing 90 percent of breast cancers in men.

Practically speaking, from a drug treatment point of view, there are three major types of breast cancer. They differ in terms of the best drugs to treat them, so it's critically important for a pathologist to be as precise as possible in his or her diagnosis.

ER/PR-Positive (ER/PR+) Breast Cancer

This is the most common category of breast cancer, affecting about 82 percent of men with the disease. ER stands for estrogen receptor, and PR stands for progesterone receptor.

HER2-Positive (HER2+) Breast Cancer

About 14 percent of men with breast cancers are in this category. HER2 stands for human epidermal growth factor receptor number 2. The HER2 gene is amplified in this form of breast cancer and acts like an accelerator for cancer cells.

---

17. *http://www.blabbermouth.net/news/original-kiss-drummer-peter-criss-says-early-breast-cancer-detec tion-saved-his-life/#8RqBgjoMkweqzElD.99*

Triple-Negative Breast Cancer (TNBC)

This type of cancer lacks the three biomarkers (ER/PR and HER2) that define the other two types. About 4 percent of male breast cancers are in this category.

Detecting these types using special tests in a medical laboratory is a process called companion diagnostics. Companion refers to the fact that precision medicine drugs—aka targeted therapies—to treat each type go hand in hand with the presence or absence of their companion biomarkers, which are often cellular proteins called receptors.

———————————— MY JOURNEY ————————————

It's just plain weird to get what most people call a "woman's disease." I'm an average guy who grew up thinking that breasts were a female thing—something to look at and admire and want to touch and feel. I think I'm pretty typical in this respect, and when I got diagnosed with breast cancer, it was very confusing and forced me to let go of many preconceived notions I had held in that respect.

My first challenge, besides all the physical stuff, was to get rid of the notion that I was any less of a man because I had lost a breast. It was hard to tell people because I couldn't help thinking I saw these raised eyebrows whenever I said the words "breast cancer," as if I was suddenly less of a man because I was dealing with something that's supposed to happen only to women. I now can understand much better what it must be like for a woman to go through this. Except that there is an enormous community of people ready to help women with breast cancer, unlike for men, where it is still a subject most people—including men—know nothing and don't even have it on their radar when it comes to paying attention to their own bodies or discussing it with their doctors.

Maybe someday, in spite of the low numbers, the cancer world will up their game on this disease, because it is real and it's scary and it needs attention. It can start with men paying attention to their bodies and not relying on someone else to do it, as I was lucky enough to benefit from when my wife pointed out to my doctor that I was feeling a lump in my breast. Thank God she spoke up so that I am still alive today.

Jan (Portland, Maine)

Cell-to-Cell Communication:
Hormone and Growth Factor Receptors
as Targets of Precision Medicines

For the specialized cells in our bodies to grow and function normally, they need to "talk" to or signal one another in ways that program or reprogram what they're doing at particular times. This cell-to-cell communication is carried out by a diverse variety of substances, such as hormones, like estrogen, and growth factors that bind to specific receptors on the surfaces of cells—like locks and keys that operate on-off switches.

Both hormones and growth factors signal cells to turn certain functions on or off, like milk production in the breast. Mutations in genes that cause cancer often act by corrupting these signaling systems, which result in uncontrolled cell growth, allowing them to spread to other parts of the body in a process we refer to as *metastasizing*.

For example, HER2 is a growth factor receptor that is necessary in small amounts to maintain the health of normal breast cells. However, in HER2+ breast cancer, abnormally large amounts of HER2 are produced on the outside of cells and this drives tumor growth.

Surgical Treatments and Potential Side Effects

Most patients with breast cancer have surgery to remove the cancer. These surgeries can have multiple effects for many men that have consequences beyond the realm of their cancer treatment. Surgery types include the following:

Breast-conserving surgery aims to remove the cancer and some normal tissue around it, but not the breast itself. This type of surgery may also be called lumpectomy, partial mastectomy, segmental mastectomy, or breast-sparing surgery. While commonly used in women, this procedure is not typically used in men for three reasons: 1) there is less breast to "spare"; 2) tumors in men are generally larger and more advanced; and 3) the frequent involvement of the nipple and areola.

Total mastectomy removes the entire breast that has cancer. This is also called a simple mastectomy. Some sentinel lymph nodes (Chapter 2) may also be removed and checked for cancer spread.

Modified radical mastectomy removes the whole breast that has cancer, many of the lymph nodes under the arm, the lining over the chest muscles, and, in some cases, part of the chest wall muscles.

In *Reimagining Women's Cancers*, Chapter 5 is devoted to oncoplastic surgery and breast reconstruction, including nipple reconstruction and medical tattoos. Many of these methods are applicable to men.

After a mastectomy, the skin of the chest may feel tight. The surrounding muscles may feel stiff or weak. If muscles have been removed, other muscles will need to learn to take over for the missing muscles.

Two other potential postmastectomy complications involve the abnormal collection of fluid: seroma and lymphedema.

Seroma is a collection of serous fluid in the body where tissue has been removed by surgery. This sterile, clear to pale yellow body fluid lines the inside of body cavities. Fluid can build up under the skin close to an incision. Seromas typically occur within one to two weeks after surgery. If the fluid builds up too much, the area will look swollen and may be painful.

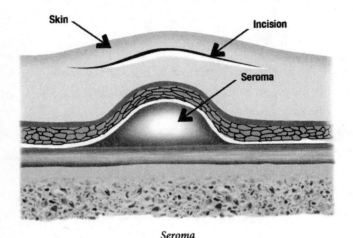

Seroma

If the seroma is small, nothing may need to be done. The body will reabsorb the excess fluid. Larger seromas are treated by removing the excess fluid with a needle and syringe. This may need to be done more than once. Pain medication, such as acetaminophen or ibuprofen, may be suggested to ease the pain.

Although it is uncommon, seromas can become infected, so watch for warning signs, including redness or warmth at the site and fever over 101.4° F, or drainage of cloudy or bloody fluid from the incision.

Lymphedema is the build-up of fluid in soft body tissue when the lymph system is damaged or blocked. It is a common problem that may be caused by cancer and its treatment. Lymphedema usually affects an arm or leg, but it can also affect other parts of the body.

Lymphedema can occur after any cancer or treatment that affects the flow of lymph through the lymph nodes, such as the removal of lymph nodes or radiation therapy. Lymphedema often occurs in breast

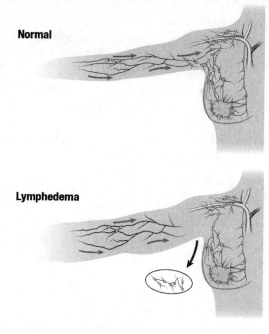

Lymphedema
©Alila Medical Media, *www.AlilaMedicalMedia.com*. Reprinted with permission.

cancer patients who have had all or part of the breast removed and axillary (underarm) lymph nodes removed.

Lymphedema may develop within days or it can occur many years after treatment. Most often it develops within three years of surgery.

Possible signs of lymphedema include the following:

- Swelling of an arm or leg, which may include fingers and toes
- A full or heavy feeling in an arm or leg
- A tight feeling in the skin
- Trouble moving a joint in the arm or leg
- Thickening of the skin, with or without skin changes, such as blisters or warts

- A feeling of tightness when wearing clothing, shoes, bracelets, watches, or rings
- Itching or burning feeling in the legs or toes
- Trouble sleeping

Radiation therapy aimed at the chest may also cause the following side effects:

- Difficulty swallowing
- Shortness of breath
- Breast or nipple soreness
- Shoulder stiffness
- Cough, fever, and fullness of the chest, which is called radiation pneumonitis and usually happens two weeks to six months after radiation therapy

Before and After Surgery: Neoadjuvant and Adjuvant Therapy

Chemotherapy may be given before surgery to shrink the tumor and reduce the amount of tissue that needs to be removed during the operation. This is called neoadjuvant therapy. Even if the surgeon removes all the cancer that is visible at the time of the surgery, some patients may be given radiation therapy, chemotherapy, or hormone therapy after surgery to kill any remaining cancer cells. Treatments given after the surgery to lower the risk that the cancer will come back are called adjuvant therapy.

Hormone Therapy and Chemotherapy

Because the large majority of male breast cancers have estrogen receptors and the tumor cells require the hormone estrogen to grow, blocking these receptors with drugs is the first line of therapy for metastatic breast cancer.

Tamoxifen (Nolvadex) is the drug mostly commonly used for this purpose. A number of other antiestrogen drugs are available and used routinely to treat female breast cancer, but many are of unproven benefit for treating male breast cancer.

Despite the effectiveness of tamoxifen in extending the lives of men with breast cancer, a large proportion of men discontinue treatment because of side effects, which include fatigue, anxiety, sleep disorders, decreased libido, and weight gain.

Chemotherapy drugs halt the growth of cancer cells by either killing the cells or stopping them from dividing. Traditional chemotherapies can have very unpleasant side effects because they tend to indiscriminately kill all rapidly dividing cells, like hair follicles and the cells lining the stomach and intestines.

Systemic chemotherapy is when drugs are given by mouth or injection and circulate throughout the entire body. This is a second line of treatment for breast cancer if and when the cancer becomes resistant to hormone therapy.

Two chemotherapy regimens that have been used to treat male breast cancer are borrowed from the treatment of breast cancer in women. The first regimen is CMF, which are the initials of the three drugs used: cyclophosphamide, methotrexate, and 5-fluorouracil. Another common regimen is FAC, which stands for 5-fluorouracil, anthracycline (daunorubicin), and cyclophosphamide. These drug regimens are given intravenously.

For more information on specific drugs, we recommend the U.S. National Library of Medicine website (*http://dailymed.nlm.nih.gov/ dailymed/*).

Targeted Therapy

Like a precision-guided smart bomb, targeted therapy uses drugs to attack specific cancer cells with minimal or manageable side effects on normal cells. As explained in Chapter 1, the drug imatinib (Gleevec) was a first-in-class drug of this kind, developed to treat a specific blood cancer. In the years since it was developed, the same principles have led to a new generation of drugs that treat a variety of solid tumors, such as lung cancer and breast cancer.

These targeted drugs come in two forms:

1. *Small molecule drugs* come in pill form or as capsules to be taken orally. They are often labeled with the suffix "ib" or "nib." These drugs block certain cancer pathways inside cancer cells. One such drug used to treat HER2+ breast cancer is lapatinib (Tykerb). Another is palbociclib (Ibrance).

2. *Monoclonal antibody drugs*, sometimes called biologics, come as liquids that are injected into the body. These drugs are labeled with the suffix "mab." They work by binding to and blocking the action of receptors on the surfaces of cancer cells.

   The following mab drugs are used to treat HER2+ breast cancer:

   • Trastuzumab (Herceptin)
   • Pertuzumab (Perjeta)
   • Ado-trastuzumab emtansine (Kadcyla), a variation of trastuzumab, which is chemically combined with a small molecule drug. This arrangement is known as an antibody-drug conjugate.

For more information on these drugs, we recommend the U.S. National Library of Medicine website *(http://dailymed.nlm.nih.gov /dailymed/)*.

Immunotherapy

Options are on the horizon for treating cancer by supporting our bodies' natural defenses and immune system. We describe this concept in Chapter 11, and some of these options have already led to next-generation treatments for several types of cancer. At the present time, there are no FDA-approved immunotherapies for breast cancer, but research into this approach may soon yield breakthroughs in the treatment of breast cancer, just as it has for other cancer types.

KEY POINTS TO REMEMBER

✓ Men can, and do, get breast cancer.

✓ About one in 1,000 men will be diagnosed with breast cancer, compared to a risk of one in eight for women.

✓ All men who develop breast cancer, at any age, are candidates for genetic counseling and testing. The information can be critical for their family members.

✓ Breast cancer in men is usually diagnosed at a later age than in women, typically around age sixty.

✓ As in women, the majority of male breast cancers are not hereditary. Men can also have hereditary breast cancer due to mutations in several genes, including BRCA2.

✓ The most common symptom is a hard, painless lump.

✓ Surgery is typically the first stage of male breast cancer treatment.

✓ Complications from surgical treatment can include seroma and lymphedema.

✓ Men who feel a lump in their breast should have it investigated!

What Cancer Cannot Do

Cancer is so limited . . .
It cannot cripple love.
It cannot shatter hope.
It cannot corrode faith.
It cannot eat away peace.

It cannot destroy confidence.

6

WHAT NO MAN WANTS TO SAY OUT LOUD: Cancer of the Penis— PeIN and Prevention

*Being the richest man in the
cemetery doesn't matter to me . . .
Going to bed at night saying we've done something
wonderful . . . that's what matters to me.*

—Steve Jobs

What Is Penile Cancer?

Cancer of the penis, also called penile cancer, is a rare and preventable disease, especially in developed nations where men are circumcised shortly after birth. Vaccination against sexually transmitted infections with human papillomavirus (HPV) is probably the best method of prevention. For those men who do develop penile cancer, new penis-preserving and reconstructive surgeries are available.

In the United States, where the rate is less than one case per 100,000 men per year, it is estimated that in 2016 about 2,000 new cases will be diagnosed, and 340 men will lose their lives from the disease.

Basic Anatomy and Function

The penis is a rod-shaped male reproductive organ that passes sperm and urine from the body. It contains two types of erectile tissue—spongy tissue with blood vessels that fill with blood to make an erection:

- *Corpora cavernosa*: The two columns of erectile tissue that form most of the penis.
- *Corpus spongiosum*: A single column of erectile tissue that forms a small portion of the penis, which surrounds the urethra (the tube through which urine and sperm pass from the body).

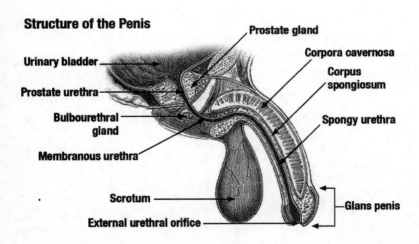

Structure of the Penis
Source: National Cancer Institute

The erectile tissue is wrapped in connective tissue and covered with skin. The glans (head of the penis) is covered with loose skin, called the foreskin.

When a man gets an erection, nerves signal the blood vessels inside the corpora cavernosa to dilate. Blood fills chambers in the spongy tissue, which expand and cause the penis to elongate and stiffen. During ejaculation, semen, which is made up of sperm and nutrient fluid, passes through and then out of the urethra. After ejaculation, nerve signals cause constriction of the penile arteries, forcing blood out of the erectile tissue, and the penis becomes soft again.

Virtually all penile carcinomas are of squamous cell origin. Squamous cells are thin, flat cells that look like fish scales and are found in the tissue that form the surface of the skin, the lining of the hollow organs of the body, and the lining of the respiratory and digestive tracts. Most penile cancers occur on the foreskin (in men who have not been circumcised) or on the glans of the penis.

—————————— MY JOURNEY ——————————

My husband was forty-eight when he died from penile cancer. He left me with two children to take care of alone. The truth is, he was too uptight to go see his doctor when he started feeling symptoms, and by the time he did visit his doctor, several months later, when it was becoming so painful he could barely get dressed, he had to have a piece of his penis removed. But it was still too late, because the cancer had already progressed. He died a few months later. My poor husband felt too ashamed to admit that there was something wrong, and all that procrastination ended up killing him. I hope other men will read this and not wait if they have any symptoms. If you can't get it together to go get checked for yourself, at least do it for your kids.

Jackie (Savannah, Georgia)

What Is PeIN? Can It Lead to Cancer?

PeIN stands for penile intraepithelial neoplasia. Epithelium refers to the outer layer of cells that line the surface of the penis. Intraepithelial means that the disease is in this layer of cells and hasn't spread beyond it. Neoplasia means "new growth" and refers to an abnormal growth of tissue in both cancer and precancerous conditions. PeIN is a precancerous condition involving an abnormal growth of tissue in the outer layer of cells of the penis and is associated with chronic HPV infection (described in the next section). If untreated, it can sometimes progress to cancer.

HPV and How It Causes Cancer

One-third to one-half of penile cancer cases are associated with persistent infection with HPV, which is a group of more than 150 related viruses. More than forty of these viruses can be easily spread through direct skin-to-skin contact during vaginal, anal, and oral sex.

HPV infections are the most common sexually transmitted infections in the United States. In fact, more than half of sexually active people are infected with one or more HPV types at some point in their lives. Sexually transmitted HPVs fall into two categories: low-risk HPV and high-risk HPV.

Low-risk HPVs, which do not cause cancer, can cause skin warts—technically known as condylomata acuminata—on or around the genitals or anus. For example, HPV types 6 and 11 cause 90 percent of all genital warts.

High-risk or oncogenic HPVs can cause cancer. At least a dozen high-risk HPV types have been identified. Two of these, HPV types 16 and 18, are responsible for the majority of cancers caused by HPV.

High-risk HPV infection accounts for approximately 5 percent of all cancers worldwide. It's important to know that most high-risk HPV infections occur without any symptoms, go away within one to two years, and do not cause cancer. These transient infections may cause cytological abnormalities, or abnormal cell changes, that go away on their own. Some HPV infections, however, can last for many years. Persistent infections with high-risk HPV types can lead to more serious cytological abnormalities or lesions that, if untreated, may progress to cancer.

How High-Risk HPVs Cause Cancer

HPVs infect epithelial cells, which are organized in layers, covering the inside and outside surfaces of the body, including the skin, throat, genital tract, and anus. HPVs are not thought to enter the bloodstream. Therefore, an HPV infection in one part of the body will not cause an infection in another part of the body.

Once an HPV enters an epithelial cell, the virus begins to make proteins. Two of the proteins made by high-risk HPVs interfere with normal functions in the cell, enabling the cell to grow in an uncontrolled manner and avoid cell death.

Many times these infected cells are recognized by the immune system and eliminated. But if these infected cells are not destroyed, a persistent infection results. As the infected cells continue to grow, they may develop mutations that promote even more cell growth, leading to the formation of a high-grade lesion and, ultimately, a tumor.

Virtually all cervical cancers are caused by HPV infections, with just two HPV types, 16 and 18, responsible for about 70 percent of all cases. HPV also causes anal cancer, with about 85 percent of all cases caused by HPV. Types 16 and 18 have also been found to cause close to half of vaginal, vulvar, and penile cancers.

Other Risk Factors

A number of studies show that circumcision may help prevent infection with HPV. A circumcision is an operation in which the doctor removes part or all of the foreskin from the penis. Many boys are circumcised shortly after birth. Men who were not circumcised at birth may have a higher risk of developing penile cancer.

Other risk factors for penile cancer include the following:

- *Being age sixty or older:* The average age of a man when diagnosed is sixty-eight, and about four out of five penile cancers are diagnosed in men over age fifty-five.
- *Having phimosis:* In this condition, the foreskin of the penis becomes tight and cannot be pulled back over the glans.
- *Poor personal hygiene:* Uncircumcised men should regularly pull back their foreskin to clean under it. If they don't do this, secretions and dead skin cells can build up. This thick, waxy substance (known as smegma) can cause irritation and inflammation of the penis.
- *Multiple sexual partners:* Increases usual risks.
- *Using tobacco products:* Smoking and chewing.
- *Men with AIDS:* Have a higher risk of penile cancer, which is likely due to their weakened immune system.

———————— **MY JOURNEY** ————————

Like most men I know, I put off going to the doctor as long as I could. I had a rash under my foreskin and it hurt pulling it back, and then I started getting some smelly discharge, which grossed me out pretty good. I guess the last straw was when the area started swelling up and really started hurting, no matter what position I tried to get into.

The first procedure I had was a circumcision, which kind of freaked me out, but it helped quite a bit. My wife was relieved, that is, until my biopsy come back telling me I had cancer. I didn't even know you could get cancer in your penis. Of course, I knew you could get a whole lot of ugly stuff down there, and I had crabs once when I was a kid, but cancer? I thought at first the doc was telling me some kind of twisted joke.

I told my coworkers that I had some cancer in my hip, so when they saw me walking funny, they wouldn't get any strange ideas. I didn't tell my kids much of anything. I let their mother do that because she just knows how to talk about anything, especially medical stuff like that. I had enough trouble just dealing with the treatment. Anyway, I battled this thing on and off for a number of years. Now it appears to be finally gone. I know I'm damn lucky, because I almost waited too long in the first place. And the surgery they did to fix my penis so it still works? That's a miracle from God, I am sure of that. And now, I'm looking forward to marrying off my oldest daughter.

Raul (West Lafayette, Indiana)

Signs and Symptoms

The main symptoms of penile cancer include redness, irritation, a sore or lump on the penis, and a discharge or bleeding. These signs may be caused by other conditions, so check with your doctor if you have any concerns.

Benign conditions of the penis are noncancerous conditions that can affect the penis. Most benign conditions of the penis affect the glans (head or glans penis) and foreskin, but they can also affect the shaft. These benign conditions include the following:

- *Condyloma* (genital wart) is the most common benign condition of the penis. The growths tend to look like tiny cauliflowers and can vary greatly in size. Some can be as large as an inch or more in diameter, while others are so small that they can be seen only with a magnifying lens. Condylomas are caused by infection with some types of HPV.

- *Bowenoid papulosis* consists of small red or brown spots or patches or papules (small, raised, solid pimples). Like condyloma, Bowenoid papulosis is associated with an HPV infection and tends to occur in younger, sexually active men. Bowenoid papulosis is typically asymptomatic but can be inflamed, pruritic, or painful. When looked at under a microscope, dysplastic (abnormal) cells are seen in the surface layer of the penile skin. Most times Bowenoid papulosis doesn't cause problems and often resolves on its own in a few months. It rarely progresses to Bowen disease, another name for penile carcinoma *in situ*, in which cancer cells are found only in the top layers of the skin.

Diagnosing Penile Cancer

The following tests and procedures may be used to diagnose penile cancer:

- *Physical exam and history:* This includes checking general signs of health, including the penis for signs of disease, such as lumps or anything else that seems unusual. A history of the patient's health habits and past illnesses and treatments is also taken.

- *Biopsy:* Cells or tissues are removed and viewed under a microscope by a pathologist who checks for signs of cancer. Tissue sample is removed during one of the following procedures:

1. *Fine-needle aspiration (FNA) biopsy*: removal of tissue or fluid using a thin needle
2. *Incisional biopsy*: removal of part of lump or sample of tissue that doesn't look normal
3. *Excisional biopsy*: removal of entire lump or area of tissue that doesn't look normal

Treatment

After penile cancer has been diagnosed, tests are done to learn if cancer cells have spread within the penis or to other parts of the body. This process is called staging, which is important to know in order to plan treatment (see Chapter 1).

When diagnosed early, that is, stage 0, stage I, and stage II, penile cancer is highly curable. Curability decreases sharply for stage III and stage IV. Because of the rarity of this cancer in the United States, clinical trials specifically for penile cancer are infrequent. Patients with stage III and stage IV cancer can be candidates for phase I or II clinical trials testing new drugs, biologicals, or surgical techniques to improve local control and distant metastases.

Surgery

Surgery is the most common treatment for all stages of penile cancer. A doctor may remove the cancer using one of the following operations:

- *Mohs microsurgery* cuts the tumor from the skin in thin layers. During the surgery, the edges of the tumor and each layer of tumor removed are viewed through a microscope to check for cancer cells. Layers continue to be removed until no more cancer cells are seen. This type of surgery removes as little normal tissue as possible and is often used to remove cancer on the skin. It is also called Mohs surgery.

- *Laser surgery* uses a laser beam (a narrow beam of intense light) that acts as a knife to make bloodless cuts in tissue or to remove a surface lesion such as a tumor. It has been successfully used as a first-line therapy for premalignant and early stage lesions since the 1980s.
- *Cryosurgery* uses an instrument with liquid nitrogen. This treatment freezes and destroys abnormal tissue. It is used more commonly in the treatment of genital warts and premalignant conditions than for penile cancer.
- *Circumcision* removes all or part of the foreskin.
- *Wide local excision* removes only the cancer and some normal tissue around it.
- *Amputation* removes part of the penis or the entire organ. If part of the penis is removed, it is called a partial penectomy. If the entire penis is removed, it is a total penectomy.

Recent surgical advances have allowed for less radical, organ-sparing techniques, with more acceptable psychosexual and oncological outcomes.

Lymph nodes in the groin may also be removed during surgery. Even if the doctor removes all the cancer that can be seen at the time of the surgery, some patients may be given chemotherapy or radiation therapy after surgery to kill any remaining cancer cells. Treatment after the surgery to lower the risk that the cancer will return is called adjuvant therapy.

Radiotherapy

Radiotherapy can be used on its own or with surgery/chemotherapy. It uses high-energy X-rays or other types of radiation to kill cancer cells or keep them from growing. External radiation therapy uses a machine outside the body to send radiation toward the cancer. The entire shaft of the penis receives treatment five times a week for four weeks. The tumor and a small area around it get an additional booster dose during this time.

Internal radiation therapy, also called brachytherapy (BT), uses a radioactive substance sealed in needles, seeds, wires, or catheters that are placed directly into or near the cancer. Two common BT techniques are used in the treatment of penile cancer. In the first, a radioactive mold is placed over the penis and is worn by the patient for twelve hours a day until the total dosage is reached. In the second technique, radioactive iridium (Ir-192) in the form of a seed is placed into the penis and removed after the appropriate dosage has been received.

The main advantage is overall good cosmetic effect and penile preservation. Complications include meatal stenosis and urethral strictures, a narrowing of the opening of the urethra, pain, ulceration, and infection.

For men who have a tumor that is surgically difficult to remove and involves the lymph nodes in the groin (on one or both sides) in any way, surgery alone is rarely curative. For these men, a course of neoadjuvant chemotherapy may be advised. Neoadjuvant simply means that it is used before surgery, primarily in the hope that the tumor will shrink and become more amenable to surgical removal.

The recommended regimen for this consists of three drugs: paclitaxel, ifosfamide, and cisplatin (TIP). Chemotherapy is given for four cycles at three to four week intervals. This same regimen can also be used as adjuvant therapy.

Can Immunization Prevent Penile Cancer?

In the case of penile cancer, the answer is possibly yes. Penile cancer is one of the few cancers whose primary cause can be linked to a specific virus—HPV (human papillomavirus)—and there are now three FDA approved vaccines to prevent it: Gardasil, Gardasil 9, and Cervarix.

Like other immunizations that guard against viral infections, HPV vaccines stimulate the body to produce antibodies that, in future encounters with HPV, bind to the virus and prevent it from infecting cells. The current HPV vaccines are based on virus-like particles (VLPs) that are formed by HPV surface components. VLPs are not infectious, because they lack the virus's DNA. However, they closely resemble the natural virus, and antibodies against the VLPs are also active against the natural virus. VLPs are strongly immunogenic, which means that they induce high levels of antibody production by the body. This makes the vaccines highly effective.

HPV vaccines are very effective in preventing infection with the types of HPV they target but are most effective when they are given before any initial exposure to the virus—*before* an individual begins to engage in sexual activity. This is why the Advisory Committee on Immunization Practices (ACIP)[18] recommends that routine HPV vaccination begins at eleven or twelve years old. The series can safely be started as young as nine years of age. They also recommend vaccination of females ages thirteen through twenty-six years and of males ages thirteen through twenty-one years who have not been vaccinated previously or who have not completed the three-dose vaccination series.

All three vaccines prevent infections with HPV types 16 and 18, two high-risk HPVs that cause about 70 percent of cervical cancers and an even higher percentage of some of the other HPV-associated cancers, including cancer of the penis.

---

18. ACIP is a group of fifteen medical and public health experts that develops recommendations on how to use vaccines to control diseases in the United States.

Gardasil prevents infection with HPV types 6 and 11, which cause 90 percent of genital warts. Gardasil 9 is the newest HPV vaccine. It prevents infection with the same four HPV types as Gardasil plus five additional high-risk HPV types (31, 33, 45, 52, and 58).

The FDA has approved Gardasil and Gardasil 9 for use in females ages nine through twenty-six for the prevention of HPV-caused cervical, vulvar, vaginal, and anal cancers; precancerous cervical, vulvar, vaginal, and anal lesions; and genital warts. Gardasil and Gardasil 9 are also approved for use in males for the prevention of HPV-caused anal cancer, precancerous anal lesions, and genital warts. Gardasil is approved for use in males ages nine through twenty-six, and Gardasil 9 is approved for use in males ages nine through fifteen.

All of the HPV vaccines are designed to be administered in three shots over a six-month period. The second shot is given one or two months after the first shot. Then a third shot is given six months after the first shot.

Although HPV vaccines are safe when given to people who are already infected with HPV, the vaccines do not treat infection. They provide maximum benefit if a person receives them *before* he or she is sexually active.

As for safety, before any vaccine is licensed, the FDA must determine that it is both safe and effective. All three HPV vaccines have been tested in tens of thousands of people in the United States and many other countries. Thus far, the vaccines have not shown any serious side effects. The most common problems have been brief soreness and other local symptoms at the injection site. These problems are similar to those commonly experienced with other vaccines.

——————————— **MY JOURNEY** ———————————

I had just retired when I found a red, blotchy rash on the tip of my penis. I didn't waste any time going to my doctor, but I was still diagnosed with cancer, and they had to remove a good portion of my organ in order to save my life. Now, if anyone thinks that this didn't matter, that I was too old to still be having sex, they are totally mistaken. In fact, I was looking forward to enjoying much more of that in my retirement when I figured I would have much more time and not be so tired from working long hours on an assembly line. So this has really messed me up, in more ways than one, but the worst is having no chance to have sex like I thought I would. I am working to find other ways to feel good, but it's not easy, for me or my wife. God bless her. I'd be dead without her.

Bert (Birmingham, Alabama)

KEY POINTS TO REMEMBER

✓ Cancer of the penis is a rare condition in developed countries.

✓ One-third to one-half of cases of penile cancer are associated with human papillomavirus (HPV) infection.

✓ HPV vaccines that can prevent infection are available. They are most effective when given prior to becoming sexually active.

✓ Other risk factors include age over sixty, being uncircumcised, having phimosis, poor hygiene, smoking, and AIDS.

✓ The main symptoms include redness, irritation, a sore or lump on the penis, or discharge or bleeding.

✓ When diagnosed early, penile cancer is highly curable.

✓ Surgery is the most common treatment for penile cancer.

✓ New, less invasive surgical procedures can often avoid penis amputation and preserve sexual function.

✓ Chemotherapy may be needed before or after surgery in patients with advanced disease.

WHAT CANCER CANNOT DO

Cancer is so limited . . .
It cannot cripple love.
It cannot shatter hope.
It cannot corrode faith.
It cannot eat away peace.
It cannot destroy confidence.

It cannot kill friendship.

7

WHAT AM I DEALING WITH? Defining Short-Term Challenges of Treatment

My veins are filled, once a week with a Neapolitan carpet cleaner distilled from the Adriatic and I am as bald as an egg. However I still get around and am mean to cats.

—John Cheever, from a 1982 letter to Philip Roth,
regarding his cancer and its treatment,
from *The Letters of John Cheever*

Do Your Due Diligence

Any kind of cancer treatment can cause challenging side effects. Problems may arise when treatment designed to impact cancerous tissues also affects healthy tissues or organs. Each person undergoing a treatment regimen reacts to it in his or her individual way.

Some people experience very few side effects while others may need to endure more than were anticipated.

Several factors contribute to the side effects you may experience, including the type(s) of treatment, the amount or frequency of the treatment, your age, and any other health conditions you may already have. Most of the short-term side effects discussed in this chapter will improve after treatment has ended, although some may take weeks or months to resolve completely.

> NOTE to PATIENT:
> Before you begin any kind of treatment,
> ask your healthcare team which side effects are
> likely to present challenges. Learn about the steps you
> can take to lessen them, during—and after—treatment.

Surgery: What Are the General Risks and Side Effects?

Complications during surgery can be caused by the procedure itself; the drugs used before, during, and/or after the procedure (including the anesthesia); or any underlying disease a patient may already have. In general, the more complex the surgery, the greater the risk.

Surgical procedures today are generally safer than they have ever been. Technical advances, including less invasive, microsurgical, and robotic surgical techniques, have improved safety levels and shortened recovery time. Despite these breakthroughs, there is always a small risk to any surgical procedure. Some of these include the following:

- Bleeding
- Damage to nearby tissues, such as blood vessels or nerves

- Reactions to drugs or anesthesia used during the procedure
- Damage to other organs, such as the lungs, heart, or kidneys (more common if you already have conditions that affect these organs)

The most common post-operative problems after surgery include the following:

- *Pain:* This is normal after any surgery, and its frequency and level depends on how extensive a procedure you have had, as well as your individual pain threshold. Medications for pain relief range from acetaminophen to stronger drugs, such as codeine and morphine. Some of them are dispensed in pill form, while others may be included in a post-op IV.
- *Infections:* The most likely location is at the surgical site. Your doctor may prescribe antibiotics prophylactically or later if there are any signs of infection. They may be given by mouth or through a vein. Contracting pneumonia is possible for any patient with previously impaired lung function, such as smokers, or if pain from the procedure prevents the patient from taking deep breaths.
- *Slow recovery of other body functions:* Symptoms such as decreased bowel activity may occur after surgery due to inactivity, change in diet, and medications.

Joe Torre: Striking Out Prostate Cancer

Because heart disease runs in his family, former New York Yankee manager Joe Torre had a checkup and medical testing with his cardiologist every year. In 1999, his doctor told him that his PSA was slightly elevated and suggested a repeat.

"My PSA came back at 4.5 ng/ml," Joe said, "and my free PSA was extremely low. A biopsy that was performed shortly after came back positive. I was told that I had an aggressive cancer."

Based on the aggressiveness of the cancer and his age (fifty-eight), Torre's doctor recommended a radical prostatectomy. "My surgery proceeded without any complications and the specialist said it had been successful. In addition to getting all the cancer out, he was also able to save both nerves on the prostate that control sexual function. Back home from the hospital, I had some post-operative problems with incontinence but they cleared up very quickly."[19]

In May of that year, Torre returned to the Yankees, leading them to a second-consecutive World Series title. Torre has also become an outspoken advocate for prostate cancer education, participating in a program called Your Prostate, Your Decision.[20] The goal of the campaign is to raise awareness for prostate cancer and the new genomic tests that can help determine a cancer's level of aggressiveness.

How to Recognize an Infection

Any type of cancer treatment can cause complications, including an infection, an invasion and growth of germs in the body, such as bacteria, viruses, yeast, or other fungi. An infection can begin anywhere. It may spread throughout the body and can cause one or more of these signs:

- Fever of 100.5 °F (38 °C) or higher or chills
- Cough or sore throat
- Diarrhea
- Ear pain, headache or sinus pain, or a stiff or sore neck

19. *http://www.usrf.org/news/010815-Joe_Torre_CaP.html*
20. *http://www.myprostatecancertreatment.org/yourprostateyourdecision.aspx#.VuRmVNCaagw*

- Skin rash
- Sores or white coating in the mouth or on the tongue
- Swelling or redness, especially where a catheter enters the body
- Urine that is bloody or cloudy, or pain when urinating

NOTE to PATIENT:
Call your healthcare team if you have signs of an infection. Infections during cancer treatment can be life threatening and require urgent medical attention.

MY JOURNEY

Cancer can make you feel very lonely. It is definitely not a good idea to try to deal with everything on your own. And it's not necessary. People want to help. If you don't let them, they will feel bad, and what's the point of that? Let your family and friends be right there for you, as they probably want to be, and seek support from your church or a neighborhood group, whatever works for you. There are so many cancer support groups. It's amazing. It doesn't matter where you live, either, because you can find people dealing with similar conditions all over the Internet just waiting to listen and to help.

Scott (Boise, Idaho)

Radiation Therapy:
General Risks and Side Effects

Radiation therapy destroys cancer cells by damaging their DNA (the molecules inside cells that carry genetic information and pass it from one generation to the next). It can either damage DNA directly or create charged particles (free radicals) within the cells that, in turn, can damage the DNA. Cancer cells containing DNA that is damaged beyond repair will stop dividing and self-destruct. When the damaged cells die, they are broken down and eliminated naturally by the body.

Unfortunately, radiation therapy can also damage normal cells, leading to side effects. Doctors take this into account when planning a course of therapy. The amount of radiation that normal tissue can safely receive is known for all parts of the body. Doctors use this information to help them decide where to aim radiation most effectively.

Radiation therapy can cause both early (acute) and late (chronic) side effects. Acute side effects occur during treatment, and chronic side effects occur months or even years after treatment ends. The side effects depend on the area of the body being treated, the dose given each day (as well as the total dose received), your general medical health, as well as other treatments you may be receiving at the same time.

Acute radiation side effects are caused by damage to rapidly dividing normal cells in the area being treated. These effects can include skin irritation, dry mouth, hair loss, or urinary problems, depending upon the area of the body being treated. Most acute effects disappear after treatment ends, though some can be permanent.

Fatigue is a common side effect of radiation therapy, regardless of which part of the body is treated. Nausea with or without vomiting is common when the abdomen is treated and occurs sometimes with treatment of the brain. Medications are available to help prevent or treat nausea and vomiting during treatment.

There are two main types of radiation therapy.

1. *External beam radiation:* This therapy comes from a machine that aims radiation at your cancer. The machine is large and may be noisy. It does not touch you but can move around you, sending radiation to a part of your body from many

directions. External beam radiation therapy treats a specific part of your body. For example, if you have cancer in your breast, you will have radiation only to your chest, not to your whole body.

2. *Internal radiation:* This therapy is distinguished by having a source of radiation put inside your body. The radiation source can be solid or liquid. Internal radiation therapy with a solid source is called brachytherapy. In this type of treatment, radiation in the form of seeds, ribbons, or capsules is placed into your body in or near the cancer. You receive liquid radiation through an IV line, which allows the liquid to travel throughout your body, seeking out and killing cancer cells.

——————————————— **MY JOURNEY** ———————————————

I had radiotherapy, which caused damage to my rectum. My anus was inflamed for many months, so I had to make sure that my bowels stayed as regular as possible. Any diversion from a steady, calm diet played havoc with my digestive system. Instead of possibly just going once or twice a day, I often had to go three times a day, but at least the first time happened right away when I woke up, so I got that over with and only had to face another trip or two. I'm telling you, each time I had to go was an ordeal.

Tom (Fargo, North Dakota)

Chemotherapy: General Risks and Side Effects

Like radiation therapy, chemotherapy works by stopping or slowing the growth of cancer cells, which grow and divide quickly. But it can also harm healthy cells that divide quickly, including cells in your skin, hair, nails, the lining of your digestive system, and your blood cells.

Damage to healthy cells is the cause of side effects. Most side effects improve or go away after chemotherapy is over. Common short-term side effects of chemotherapy include the following:

- *Hair loss:* Although it may be most noticeable when the hair on your head falls out, hair loss from chemotherapy can occur all over the body, including the eyelashes and eyebrows.
- *Nausea and vomiting:* Anti-nausea drugs are often given to mitigate these side effects.
- *Nail weakness:* The nails may become brittle, break easily, or develop ridges in them.
- *Pain:* Some chemotherapy can cause temporary nerve damage, which presents itself as burning or shooting pain. The specific symptoms will depend on which peripheral nerves (sensory, motor, or autonomic) are affected.
- *Muscle soreness:* This can also be caused by chemotherapy and will usually go away after treatment is stopped, but it may take several weeks or months to resolve.
- *Mouth pain and sore throat* (mucositis/stomatitis): Chemotherapy causes irritation of the lining of the mouth and throat, making it difficult to eat and swallow.
- *Fatigue/tiredness:* This can happen randomly and not always corresponding with treatment.
- *Constipation/diarrhea*: It may be isolated or may become chronic.
- *Anemia:* This refers to a low red blood cell count. It can be manifested as fatigue, shortness of breath, and paleness.
- *Leukopenia and neutropenia:* Both refer to a low white blood cell count. It can increase your risk of infection or make you subject to infections that healthy people don't normally get.

• *Increased bruising:* This is usually due to low platelet counts.

Scott Hamilton:
A Light at the End of the Tunnel

As discussed in Chapter 4, Olympic figure skating gold medalist Scott Hamilton was diagnosed with stage III testicular cancer in 1997. His aggressive chemotherapy regimen was difficult, as he told *Coping with Cancer.*[21] "My third round of chemo was depressing because I didn't have any energy, I felt nauseous, I felt bloated, I didn't have any hair, my body had changed and I knew I wasn't going to get back to skating for quite some time. My whole life had changed so drastically that it was depressing."

Setting short-term goals helped Hamilton get through treatment. "On the last day of my third round of chemo, I realized I only had to go through this one more time. I'm convinced that you can do anything if you know you never have to do it again, so going into the fourth round of chemo, I put out my arm and said, 'Hook me up. Let's go. Let's get these five days behind me, and let's get to getting well. Let's make sure there's no more cancer in me and that whatever was in there is dead enough that we can just take it out surgically and I can get back to my life.' Once you see the light at the end of the tunnel, things get a little bit easier."

Symptoms of Peripheral Neuropathy

Neuropathy refers to nerve disease or damage. Peripheral nerves send signals to the brain through the spinal cord, such as "my feet are cold" or "stand up." Any damage to this communication system may cause a person to experience compromised movement and feeling.

---

21. *http://copingmag.com/cwc/index.php/celebrities/celebrity_article/scott_hamilton*

According to the National Institute of Neurological Disorders and Strike (part of the NIH), approximately 20 million people in the United States experience some form of peripheral neuropathy, a condition that develops as a result of damage to the peripheral nervous system, which certain cancer treatments can trigger.

Damage to sensory nerves—those that help you feel pain, heat, cold, and pressure—may cause a variety of side effects, including tingling, numbness, or a pins-and-needles feeling in your feet and hands that may spread to your legs and arms; an inability to feel hot or cold sensations; or an inability to feel pain, such as from a cut or sore on your foot.

Damage to motor nerves—those that help your muscles move— can cause weak or achy muscles, which may cause you to lose your balance or trip easily. It may also be difficult to button shirts or open jars. This side effect may also make muscles twitch/cramp, and if muscles aren't used regularly, it can lead to a condition called muscle wasting or atrophy, in which muscles become thin and weak. If your chest or throat muscles are affected, this can become especially serious if it creates difficulties in swallowing or breathing.

Damage to autonomic nerves—those that control functions such as blood pressure, digestion, heart rate, temperature, and urination— can cause digestive changes (such as constipation or diarrhea), dizziness or faintness (due to low blood pressure), sexual problems (men may be unable to get an erection and women may not reach orgasm), sweating problems (either too much or too little), and/or urination problems, such as leaking urine or difficulty emptying your bladder.

Wade Hayes: The Effects of Neuropathy

Country singer Wade Hayes burst onto the scene in 1994 with his debut album *Old Enough to Know Better*. Its title track, along with three more singles from the album, all reached the Top Ten on the Billboard Country charts.

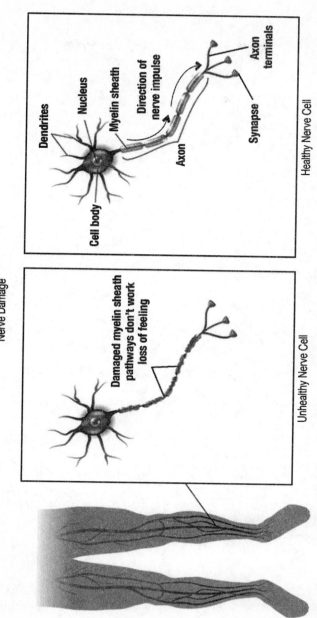

Peripheral Neuropathy
Source: © Gunita (*Dreamstime.com*)

In 2011, while touring with fellow country artist Randy Owen, Wade suddenly experienced severe abdominal pain and profuse bleeding. Although he rallied sufficiently to do the show, he saw his doctor afterward, who recommended a colonoscopy. The procedure found an orange-sized tumor in his large intestine. The diagnosis was stage IV colon cancer because the cancer had already spread to his liver, lymph nodes, and diaphragm. Wade underwent a lengthy surgery followed by chemotherapy.

Two years later, Wade faced cancer again, this time in his lymph nodes. "They opened me up from stem to stern, literally," Wade told *Country Weekly*.[22] "They had to take a big part of my large intestine, most of my liver, part of my diaphragm out, lymph nodes, and I've had several small surgeries on my liver to get it repaired enough to work correctly."

Although his cancer treatment was ultimately successful, Wade still had to deal with the side effects of that treatment. When asked by *Coping with Cancer*[23] what the biggest challenge he faced with cancer was, Wade said, "Neuropathy is the one that stands out in my mind. It's a condition where the nerve endings in your hands and feet are damaged. If you touch anything that isn't room temperature, it's very uncomfortable. You can't feel things, but you've got this strange tingling yet numb sensation. I play guitar for a living, but I couldn't feel where my fingers were on the neck of my guitar. You have to be pretty dexterous to play guitar with any accuracy, so it was difficult. It took about a year to get my dexterity back, but my hands are fine now. I still feel the effects in my feet, but fortunately, I don't play with my feet."

---

22. *http://www.countryweekly.com/news/wade-hayes-describes-second-bout-cancer*
23. *http://copingmag.com/cwc/index.php/celebrities/celebrity_article/wade_hayes*

NOTE to PATIENT:
If any of these side effects appear, inform your doctor!
Don't wait until they become unmanageable.
There are no stupid questions!

KEY POINTS TO REMEMBER

✓ Any kind of cancer treatment can cause challenging side effects.

✓ Most short-term side effects improve after treatment has ended, although some may take weeks or months to resolve completely.

✓ Before you begin any kind of treatment, ask your healthcare team which side effects are likely to present challenges. Learn about the steps you can take to lessen them, during—and after—treatment.

✓ Surgical procedures today are generally safer than they have ever been.

✓ Any type of cancer treatment can cause complications, including an infection—an invasion and growth of germs in the body, such as bacteria, viruses, yeast, or other fungi.

✓ Call your healthcare team if you have signs of an infection. They can become life threatening and require urgent medical attention.

✓ Fatigue is a common side effect of radiation therapy.

✓ Neuropathy refers to nerve disease or damage.

✓ If side effects appear, inform your doctor! Don't wait until they become unmanageable.

✓ There are no stupid questions!

WHAT CANCER CANNOT DO

Cancer is so limited . . .
It cannot cripple love.
It cannot shatter hope.
It cannot corrode faith.
It cannot eat away peace.
It cannot destroy confidence.
It cannot kill friendship.

It cannot shut out memories.

8 WHO HAVE I BECOME? Defining Long-Term Challenges of Cancer Survivorship

*Cancer can take away all of my physical abilities.
It cannot touch my mind, it cannot touch my
heart, and it cannot touch my soul.*

—Jim Valvano

What Does It Mean to Be a Survivor?

You've finished your treatments and have been given the "all clear" from your doctor. But, like many cancer patients, you may experience lingering or even new side effects, apart from the surgical scars. This chapter discusses some of the long-term complications and risks after treatment. We'll see how a number of people are dealing with these challenges. For example, Joe Andruzzi, three-time Super Bowl winner, went from being a highly motivated athlete to a temporary shell of his former self after being diagnosed with non-Hodgkin Burkitt lymphoma, and before regaining his health. Decorated Army veteran and former U.S. Senator Bob Dole ignored advice to keep his prostate cancer a secret and talked openly during multiple television appearances about his successful surgery and subsequent struggles with erectile dysfunction, prompting a slew of responses from men (and women) all across the country who thanked him for speaking out on the subject. Harry Belafonte, the legendary singer, songwriter, actor, and social activist, has also openly discussed prostate cancer and its conversational taboos: incontinence and impotence. And British actor Pete Postlethwaite fathered a daughter after being treated for testicular cancer.

So what does it really mean to be a survivor?

Most people define it as someone who has overcome something, who has reached the other side of what may be the most difficult journey of their lives. Each individual will see the process differently and vary on how they identify with the word, especially when determining when they become a survivor and how long that status applies. Since we can't foresee the future, and the concept of survivorship is not an exact science, we can only suggest that each patient approach these long-term challenges one day at a time.

Since this chapter explores an assortment of long-term effects—physical, psychological, and emotional—of cancer treatments, let's begin at the top, with "mission control."

―――――――――――― **MY JOURNEY** ――――――――――――

When my treatment ended, I was lost for quite some time, still overcome by all the emotional fatigue I had endured on this roller coaster ride. For months I had only focused on getting through each day of treatment and the effects that stuck around until the next cycle began all over again. I felt like I could never get ahead of it, not even for a day. So even when I was eventually declared cancer-free, it took me a long, long time to stop thinking about death and dying and accept the fact—the real scientific fact—that I had a lot to live for right here and now.

Bruce (New York, New York)

Chemo Brain:
When Thoughts and Feelings Run Amok

According to the National Cancer Institute, one in four people with cancer reports memory and attention problems after chemotherapy. Doctors call this phenomenon chemotherapy-related cognitive dysfunction, which is commonly referred to as chemo brain.

Many survivors describe it as a "brain fog," which can lead to problems with paying attention, trouble finding the right words, difficulty remembering new things, trouble multitasking, memory lapses, and taking longer to do things due to disorganized, slower thinking and mental processing.

These effects can begin soon after treatment ends, or they may not appear until much later. They don't always go away. If a person is older, it can be hard to tell whether these changes in memory and concentration are a result of treatment or of the aging process. Either way, some feel they just can't focus as they once did.

Research is exploring why some people develop problems with memory and concentration while others don't. It seems that people who have had chemotherapy or have had radiation to the head area are at higher risk for these problems. People who had high doses of chemotherapy may have memory problems, but even those who had standard doses have reported memory changes.

Although chemo brain was first identified and named by breast cancer survivors, research now suggests that the same constellation of symptoms also affects survivors of other cancers.

It may not be only the cancer treatment that causes chemo brain. Dr. Tim Ahles, who studies chemo brain at Memorial Sloan-Kettering Cancer Center in New York City, explains that some patients tested before starting treatment may have cognitive problems. He suggests, "Aspects of cancer biology may influence cognitive functioning, or that there are as-yet-unidentified shared risk factors for mild cognitive changes and the development of cancer. It's more complicated than chemotherapy. Almost no one who is treated for cancer receives only chemotherapy. Other aspects of treatment may be equally important to understanding changes in cognitive functioning."[24]

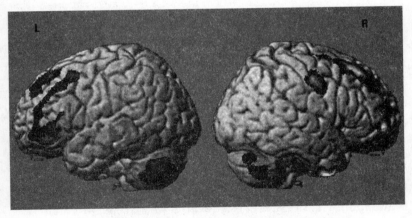

Chemo Brain. An MRI scan shows decreases in gray matter in the brain's bilateral frontal lobes and cerebellum and right temporal lobe after one month of chemotherapy.
Source: Brenna C. McDonald (used with permission)

Studies have been done using something called functional magnetic resonance imaging (fMRI), a technology that measures brain activity

---

24. *http://www.cancer.gov/about-cancer/treatment/research/understanding-chemobrain*

by detecting changes associated with blood flow. This technique relies on the fact that cerebral blood flow and neuronal activation are coupled. When an area of the brain is in use, blood flow to that region also increases. Using this method, researchers have identified structural brain abnormalities in patients treated with chemotherapy.

In another study, this time using positron emission tomography (PET) imaging, breast cancer survivors who had received chemotherapy during the previous five to ten years used more of their brains to perform a short-term memory task than control subjects who had never received chemotherapy—a sign that cancer survivors' brains have to work harder to complete the task.

Dr. Ahles, along with colleagues at Dartmouth Medical School, suggests that a form, or allele, of the APOE gene, called ε4, may be a genetic marker for increased vulnerability to chemo brain. This marker is also associated with increased risk for Alzheimer's disease. They looked at a large number of long-term breast and lymphoma survivors and found that participants who had at least one ε4 allele had significantly lower scores on standard tests of visual memory and spatial ability as well as a tendency toward lower scores on psychomotor functioning than subjects who did not carry this allele.

Dr. Patricia Ganz and her colleagues at UCLA's Jonsson Comprehensive Cancer Center suspect that uncontrolled inflammation may be a cause of chemo brain. "Many of the patients in our breast cancer survivorship program who have cognitive complaints also have fatigue, sleep disturbance, or depression," she said. "Our hypothesis is that small differences (called polymorphisms) in genes that regulate the immune system render some patients more vulnerable to this constellation of symptoms."

Many cancer treatments, including surgery, radiation, chemotherapy, and immunotherapy, can increase inflammation, Dr. Ganz added, which may not resolve after treatment ends.

Research on treatments for chemo brain is still in its very early stages. Dr. Ganz is beginning a pilot study of rehabilitation strategies for affected breast cancer survivors. Some evidence suggests that medications that stimulate the central nervous system, such as Adderall, a combination of dextroamphetamine and amphetamine, may moderate adverse cognitive effects.

For additional methods focused on managing chemo brain symptoms, please see the section "Memory and Concentration Problems" in Chapter 9.

Joe Andruzzi: Tackling Cancer's Impact

As an offensive lineman who won three Super Bowl rings with the New England Patriots, Joe Andruzzi was used to being knocked around—a lot. But nothing quite prepared him for the jolt he was about to receive in May 2007.

"I had just finished my tenth year in the NFL, and was ready to train and show people I still had something in the tank, because you get old really fast in the NFL. But I just wasn't feeling right. I went to the doctor, had a CT scan, and I found out I had a large mass wrapped around my colon. I went through an abundance of tests and was diagnosed with non-Hodgkin Burkitt lymphoma."[25]

Andruzzi underwent an aggressive course of chemotherapy, spending over three months at Dana-Farber Cancer Institute and Brigham and Women's Hospital in Boston. But Joe says he doesn't recall much of that time. "I spent more than fifty days in the hospital during three months of intensive chemotherapy. I don't remember much because of chemo brain, but I vaguely recall my wife Jen yelling at me to get

---

25. *http://blog.dana-farber.org/insight/2015/06/super-bowl-champion-joe-andruzzi-shares-his-cancer-experience/*

out of bed and walk around. But I just didn't want to move. I don't remember ever being like that. I had always been active, whether with football or just with my kids."

Joe spent the next year at home recuperating. But not being able to play the game he loved depressed him. "I had a deep depression for months. I finished treatment as football season started, and for the first time in ten or twenty years, I didn't know what I should be doing at that time of year. I didn't want to leave the house. It was a day-to-day process. You're going to have your ups and downs, but what matters is how you bounce back from being down."

When he did finally get up for good, his family founded the Joe Andruzzi Foundation, which is committed to "tackling" cancer's impact by providing financial assistance for patients and their families as well as funding pediatric brain cancer research.

Emotional Distress and Depression

For some, dealing with cancer can lead to serious depression and emotional distress. These feelings may be strongest during the first year after diagnosis, and they can manifest themselves in a variety of physical ways.

One of the most common residual effects of any cancer experience is a fear of recurrence. After cancer treatment ends, many people are afraid that they still have cancer or that it will come back. These fears are normal. For some people, talking to a counselor or joining a support group can be helpful. Your healthcare provider may be able to help you find a counselor or support group. Others may choose to seek other therapeutic options, including art therapy, expressive writing classes or journal clubs, or joining a theater group of survivors.

Volunteering at the cancer center where you were treated may also be helpful. There's nothing more hopeful for a patient in the midst of a difficult treatment protocol than to see someone else who is surviving and thriving after going through the same thing. And providing that optimism may also offer you the positive boost you may need from time to time.

MY JOURNEY

I'm not bummed out. I'm not sad. I'm depressed. I was bummed when I got diagnosed and had to deal with feeling crappy through treatment. But beating cancer was also a rush, and I think the adrenaline rush of being challenged as a patient is what carried me through to the other side.

But now that I'm here, supposedly healthy, I feel like I'm a prisoner to the haunting prospect of the cancer returning. My own mortality is screaming at me every day, even though I probably won't die from this disease. I'm tired most of the time, worn out from the worry of return, exhausted from trying to be the man I was before because I have no idea who I am now. My shrink says it's normal, that the fog will eventually lift. I guess I pay her to say positive things like that so maybe I should try to believe them.

Rick (Roanoke, Virginia)

The Extra Burden on Men

Men diagnosed with cancer are at increased risk for both depression and anxiety. This seems to be especially true when they are dealing with sexual/urinary side effects. Although it is normal for a patient to experience lows when dealing with potentially life-threatening conditions, such as cancer, depression goes beyond this, with symptoms that interfere with daily functioning. They may include some of the following:

- Persistent sad or anxious feelings
- Feelings of hopelessness
- Feelings of guilt, worthlessness, and/or helplessness
- Irritability, restlessness
- Loss of interest in activities or hobbies once considered pleasurable, including sex
- Fatigue and decreased energy
- Difficulty concentrating and memory problems
- Insomnia or excessive sleeping
- Overeating or loss of appetite
- Thoughts of suicide/suicide attempts

This list is daunting. Depression can be a life-threatening condition and should be evaluated by a physician or mental healthcare provider. Treatments include medications, cognitive behavioral therapy (a form of talk therapy), or a combination of both.

Studies have shown that there is an increased risk of suicide in men who have been diagnosed with prostate cancer or testicular cancer. A 2013 study[26] of men who had been diagnosed with prostate cancer showed a moderate increase in the risk of suicide. This increase was seen not only in patients with advanced disease but also in men with low-risk cancer. Likewise, a study by Beard[27] of over 9,000 men and colleagues treated with stage I testicular cancer demonstrated "significant suicide excesses in Stage I seminoma, which persisted for ten years after diagnosis. This finding is especially disturbing in view of the otherwise excellent prognosis for these patients."

Here is the bottom line: Men who are diagnosed and treated for cancer have an increased risk of anxiety and depression, which can significantly impact their lives, regardless of their prognosis. If you

26. http://www.ncbi.nlm.nih.gov/pubmed?term=23337463
27. http://www.ncbi.nlm.nih.gov/pmc/articles/PMC4480368/

have symptoms of depression or anxiety, speak to your physician or a mental healthcare provider. Many effective treatment options are available for you.

> NOTE to PATIENT:
> Depression is real and can be treated.

Insomnia

Whether it's anxiety, lack of quality sleep, or fluctuations in diet and exercise, any of us can experience challenges in getting adequate sleep, which can occur from the normal stressors of everyday life.

But a diagnosis of cancer can compound these normal tendencies, easily leading to insomnia if we are not careful. This can be especially troublesome because when cancer is present, our bodies naturally become more sensitive and vulnerable, and it becomes increasingly important that we get adequate sleep not only to heal physically but to give our minds and hearts the chance to enjoy a quality rest.

Medications are often used to treat insomnia in people without cancer, yet only a few studies show that they reduce insomnia specifically related to cancer treatment.

Here are some other things you can do to get a better night's sleep:

- Keep a regular schedule and avoid napping during the day
- Avoid spicy foods, caffeine, and alcohol before bedtime
- Sleep in a dark, quiet place
- Reduce tension with meditation or other relaxation techniques
- Avoid excessive TV or computer use in bed

MY JOURNEY

Cancer has really slapped me upside my head, but it's also had a wicked effect on my family and friends, not to mention my career. Every time I've had a bad day, leaving me in a bad or even foul mood, it's affected everyone else in my life. I apologize all the time, and everyone seems understanding enough, but I know that my cancer is taking a toll on them, too. I'm no fun to be around when I feel sick and scared and just plain pissed that I have to deal with this for what seems like forever. I'm trying hard not to be a jerk, but I'm sure I'm failing plenty, and I hope people will stick by me because I don't think I could make it through all of this alone.

Stephen (King of Prussia, Pennsylvania)

Gastrointestinal Disorders

Radiation therapy (RT) used to treat both prostate and testicular cancer has been associated with early *and* late toxicity in the gastrointestinal tract. Men treated with RT for testicular cancer have an increased risk of ulcers in the stomach or duodenum (the first part of the small intestine). Symptoms include bloating, heartburn, nausea or vomiting, and a gnawing or burning pain in the middle or upper stomach, which can occur between meals or at night.

In prostate cancer patients, RT can cause proctitis, inflammation of the rectum and anus, or enteritis, inflammation of the colon. Symptoms include abdominal cramps, increased frequency of bowel movements, diarrhea, sensations of having to go urgently, and tenesmus, a continual or recurrent feeling that you need to empty your bowels. Occasionally, you may pass bright red blood in the stools. These symptoms can be treated with a combination of therapies, including dietary changes to bulk up the stools, exercises to improve the tone of the pelvic floor muscles, and medications, such as antidiarrheals.

A Battle to Breathe

One of the most serious complications from chemotherapy in testicular cancer patients is lung damage caused by two particular drugs.

Bleomycin can cause pneumonitis (inflammation of the lungs) and pulmonary fibrosis (PF), a disease in which inflammation in the lungs causes fibrosis, a thickening and scarring of the delicate lung tissue, rendering it unable to exchange oxygen. The primary symptoms are shortness of breath and a dry, hacking cough, although over time other symptoms may also appear, including fatigue, weight loss, and rapid, shallow breathing.

Damage to the lungs is cumulative and increases with each new course of bleomycin. Short-term lung effects (within the first three years of treatment) occur in almost half of patients, but, fortunately, these are usually mild, self-limited, and do not cause long-term impairment of lung function. Only about 1 percent of patients treated with bleomycin (usually along with etoposide and cisplatin) will develop pulmonary fibrosis severe enough to cause death.

Cisplatin can also cause late impairment of lung function in patients treated with high cumulative doses of the drug. This can happen up to ten or more years after the completion of treatment and should be considered in long-term survivors with lung symptoms.

Matters of the Heart

Nowadays, more than at any time in our history, people are living longer after a diagnosis of cancer, thanks in part to new therapies and strategies for treatment. But some of the same protocols that help people survive cancer may also damage the heart and lead to cardiovascular problems, including hypertension (high blood pressure), cardiac arrhythmia (heart rhythm problems), and heart failure.

In recent years, the evidence of cardiotoxicities has grown. Investigators from the fields of oncology and cardiology have come together to investigate the biology of these effects and search for ways to prevent, manage, and possibly reverse them. These collaborations have created an entirely new discipline, known as cardio-oncology.

MY JOURNEY

I've been receiving androgen deprivation therapy to treat my prostate cancer. I'm not sure what it really even does, but I trust my medical team. They've been great. That being said, they explained to me that this therapy can work wonders for patients with prostate cancer, but that it might also boost my chances of developing diabetes or having a heart attack or a stroke. They're still figuring out if I'm a likely target for any of that, but, meanwhile, I'm starting to wonder if I should investigate some other options. I mean, what's the point of curing my cancer if I'm going to end up croaking from a heart attack?

Nigel (Boca Raton, Florida)

What Is Cardiotoxicity?

The National Cancer Institute defines this term as the "toxicity that affects the heart." This includes not only a direct effect of the drug on the heart but also its effect on peripheral blood vessels due to altered blood flow dynamics or from thrombotic (blood clot) events.

Cardiotoxicity can be manifested in a number of ways:

- *Cardiomyopathy:* The muscles of the heart are weakened and are unable to pump as hard or efficiently as previously.
- *Heart failure:* A condition in which the heart can't pump enough blood to meet the body's needs. In some cases, the heart can't fill with enough blood. In other cases, the heart can't pump blood to the rest of the body with enough force. The most common signs and symptoms of heart failure are shortness of breath or trouble breathing; fatigue (tiredness); and swelling in the ankles, feet, legs, abdomen, and veins in the neck.
- *Arrhythmias:* Changes in the rhythm of the heartbeat, either faster or slower than usual.
- *Pericarditis:* A condition in which the membrane around the heart is inflamed. This sac is called the pericardium. The most common sign of pericarditis is chest pain. Other symptoms are weakness, palpitations, trouble breathing, and coughing.
- *Thromboembolism:* This refers to blood clots that form in a vein deep in the body, known as deep vein thromboses (DVTs). They occur when blood thickens and clumps together. Although DVTs can occur anywhere in the body, most deep vein blood clots occur in the lower leg or thigh. A blood clot in a deep vein can break off and travel through the bloodstream. The loose clot is called an embolus. It can travel to an artery in the lungs and block blood flow. This condition is called pulmonary embolism, or PE.

Cancer Drugs Can Cause Cardiotoxicity

Anthracycline drugs (such as daunorubicin, doxorubicin, and epirubicin) are used to treat many types of cancer. They work by damaging the DNA in cancer cells, causing them to die. Anthracyclines can cause heart failure, acute myocarditis (inflammation of the heart muscle), or abnormal heart rhythms.

5-Fluorouracil (5-FU), which is used to treat cancers of the breast, colon, rectum, stomach, and pancreas, interferes with cancer cells' ability to make DNA. 5-FU can cause angina-like chest pain, heart failure, and cardiogenic shock, a condition in which the heart suddenly can't pump enough blood to meet the body's needs, myocardial infarction (heart attack), and even sudden death.

Cyclophosphamide (CTX) is used to treat many types of cancer. CTX can cause neuro-hormonal changes, which can push heart dysfunction toward clinical heart failure. It can also cause the mitral valve to become leaky (mitral regurgitation).

Checking the Heart Before Treatment

Three factors must be considered in any cancer patient before dealing with the potential cardiotoxic effect of treatment:

1. Detecting patients at the highest risk
2. Developing preventive strategies
3. Early treatment of cardiotoxicity if and when it does appear

Patients with preexisting medical conditions, such as high blood pressure, cardiovascular disease, diabetes, and abnormal cholesterol profiles, may all be at higher risk of cardiotoxic effects from chemotherapy/radiation therapy, and medical management of those conditions may be needed before treatment is started.

It is recommended that all patients undergoing chemotherapy receive a pretreatment heart evaluation, which would assess any preexisting conditions and act as a baseline of heart function. This should start with a personal and family medical history as well as a physical exam, including blood pressure measurement. The most frequently used procedure—and most effective approach—to monitoring heart function is an echocardiogram (EKG), a noninvasive technique using sound waves, which can detect any arrhythmias. Research is currently assessing whether certain blood tests that can detect damage to heart muscle cells will be reliable methods to follow potential cardiotoxicity.

Specific guidelines for follow-up testing have not yet been developed; however, periodic reevaluation of heart function is important to assure the best cardiac outcomes for the ever-increasing number of long-term cancer survivors.

Chemoprevention of Cardiotoxicity

Several clinical trials are exploring new strategies for preventing or reducing damaging cardiovascular changes induced by cancer treatments. An NCI-sponsored study, for instance, will investigate whether carvedilol, a type of drug known as a beta-blocker, can prevent, or possibly reverse, damage to the heart among young adults who received high-dose anthracyclines.

In May 1995, the FDA approved dexrazoxane hydrochloride for injection (Zinecard) as a treatment to reduce the incidence and severity of cardiomyopathy associated with doxorubicin administration in certain breast cancer patients.

Another clinical trial, sponsored by NHLBI and NCI, is testing whether a statin medication, which is commonly used to treat high cholesterol, can help prevent the cardiotoxic effects of some breast cancer treatments. The Preventing Anthracycline Cardiovascular Toxicity with Statins (PREVENT)[28] trial will investigate whether the use of atorvastatin can help reduce or prevent cardiotoxicity among patients with breast cancer and lymphoma receiving anthracycline treatment.

The identification of other heart protective agents to prevent cardiotoxicity of chemotherapeutic drugs is a high priority for cardio-oncologists.

---

28. *https://clinicaltrials.gov/ct2/show/NCT01988571*

MY JOURNEY

Luckily, I started with two balls, so when I lost one to testicular cancer I was still able to function. Barely. I had so many gastrointestinal side effects, it drove me nuts. My doctors were constantly worried about infections and blood clots from the treatments. And let's not even discuss the potential for heart problems. I mean, I had two balls to start, but only one heart, and all that poison in the drugs I was treated with supposedly compromised my heart's ability to operate at its optimum. So fingers crossed for that, like for the next thirty or forty years, I hope.

Doug (Austin, Texas)

Sexual Dysfunction

For most men considering treatment for prostate, testicular, and penile cancers, the prospect of sexual dysfunction is one of their greatest fears. Dysfunction can be caused by both physical and psychosocial factors, including anxiety, depression, and partner-relationship issues.

Erectile dysfunction (ED), also known as impotence, is the most common side effect in men treated for prostate cancer. Surgery, radiation therapy, and/or chemotherapy can cause erectile dysfunction. Even with the most careful nerve-sparing surgical procedures, nearly all men treated for prostate cancer will have some degree of erectile dysfunction for the first few months following treatment.

As discussed in Chapter 6, to get an erection, nerves signal the blood vessels inside the corpora cavernosa to dilate. Blood fills chambers in the spongy tissue, which expands and causes the penis to elongate and stiffen. These nerves are very delicate and lie next to some of the blood vessels that supply the prostate. Even if they are not damaged during surgery, stretching of the nerve can cause temporary dysfunction.

According to the Prostate Cancer Foundation, "Within one year after treatment, nearly all men with intact nerves will see a substantial improvement. By this point, about 40 to 50 percent of men who undergo nerve-sparing prostatectomy will have returned to their pre-treatment function, and after two years, about 30 to 60 percent will have returned to pre-treatment function."[29]

For men who have undergone radiation therapy, the incidence of impotence is lower, but they tend not to improve as much over time and in some cases even worsen. The incidence is 25 to 50 percent for men who undergo brachytherapy and nearly 50 percent for those with external radiotherapy.

The Prostate Cancer Foundation also reports, "Men who undergo procedures that are not designed to minimize side effects and/or those whose treatments are administered by physicians who are not proficient in the procedures will fare worse. In addition, men with other diseases or disorders that impair their ability to maintain an erection, such as diabetes or vascular problems, will have a more difficult time returning to pre-treatment function."

Bob Dole: Telling It Like It Is

Robert Joseph "Bob" Dole has a long and distinguished history of public service. He served in the Army during WWII, and was badly wounded by German machine-gun fire, sustaining injuries to his upper back and right arm. He was decorated three times: two Purple Hearts for his injuries and the Bronze Star for his attempt to assist a downed radioman. He went on to represent the state of Kansas in the House of Representative from 1961 to 1969 and in the Senate from 1969 to 1996. He served as both Senate minority and majority leader. He was the vice-presidential nominee during President Gerald Ford's

---

29. *http://www.pcf.org/site/c.leJRIROrEpH/b.5836625/k.75D7/Erectile_Dysfunction.htm*

unsuccessful reelection bid and the Republican nominee for president in 1996 against President Bill Clinton.

In 1991, Dole was diagnosed with prostate cancer, picked up by PSA screening done during a routine medical checkup. "This was tough news to take. Some members of my staff urged me to keep a low profile. 'Get treatment,' they said, but do it quietly. I didn't take their advice. I issued a press release and talked openly about the diagnosis, the treatment, and the prognosis when asked about it during television appearances. In doing this, I was inspired by the example of former First Lady Betty Ford, who gave hope and courage to many women by talking openly about her breast cancer."

Senator Dole was successfully treated with surgery but was left with erectile dysfunction. After speaking to his physician, he enrolled in a clinical trial for an experimental drug called sildenafil, which came to be known as Viagra. "I never really intended to talk about ED," Dole told *cancernetwork.com*, "but, last spring, I mentioned it to Larry King during a conversation in the green room before an appearance on *Larry King Live*. To my surprise, Larry asked me about it while we were on the air. I answered his question pretty candidly on national television."[30]

The responses Dole received from men all across the country who were suffering from ED (and also from women married to men with ED) surprised him. He heard from physicians who don't specialize in urology, as well as from those who do. "Almost all of the people who contacted me," Dole said, "by phone or by letter, thanked me for speaking out on the subject. They talked about the problem, about its impact on their lives and relationships, about the difficulties they had in coming forward to seek treatment. These people were encouraged

---

30. *http://www.cancernetwork.com/articles/bob-dole-talks-about-prostate-cancer-urges-health-aware ness#sthash.xFtmIXgV.dpuf*

that ED was becoming a recognized medical problem, something that could be discussed openly."

Use It or Lose It

A penile rehabilitation program is a form of physical therapy for men with erectile dysfunction. ED occurs because of damage done to the nerves, blood vessels, and the tissues of the penis during treatment for men's pelvic cancers. The longer impotence remains, the less likely it is to resolve, secondary to a number of physical changes. Chronic impotence leads to a decrease in blood flow to the erectile tissues. This, in turn, can lead to fibrosis and loss of function of the organ.

Penile rehabilitation programs (PRP) have two aims: 1) to help men recover function by keeping the erectile tissue healthy while nerves heal from surgery, and 2) to promote the earlier return of potency. Most PRPs contain one or more of several components.

Oral medications (phosphodiesterase type 5 inhibitors [PDEi]), such as Viagra, Levitra, and Cialis, improve blood flow to the penis and help keep erectile tissue healthy. One study[31] showed that men who were given daily doses of sildenafil after nerve-sparing prostate surgery had significantly higher erectile function at thirty-six and fifty-two weeks than men without treatment, and that nearly half were able to achieve spontaneous, unassisted erections compared with only 28 percent of the control group. Another study[32] found that men on daily sildenafil were five times more likely to have spontaneous, unassisted erections than those given a placebo.

Commonly reported side effects of sildenafil include headache, upset stomach, visual disturbance, and flushing. Some patients report insomnia, nosebleeds, runny nose, or congestion.

---

31. Bannowsky, et al., *BJU International*, vol.101, no. 10, 1279–1283, 2008.
32. McCullough, et al., *The Journal of Sexual Medicine*, vol. 5, no. 2, 476–484, 2008.

Penile injections, intracorporeal injection (ICI), require a patient to inject medication (alprostadil) into his penis, a vasoactive agent that increases blood flow into the cavernous sinuses, prompting an erection. This technique can be used in men who do not have a functional nervous system. Two-thirds of men treated with ICI for twelve weeks were able to have spontaneous erections at three months, compared with 20 percent of untreated men.

The most common side effect of ICI is a mild to moderate dull ache, occurring five to ten minutes after injection in about one-third of men. A small bruise or a small nodule or lump may develop at the site of the injection over time.

Suppositories (Muse) are pellets of medicine (alprostadil) that are inserted into the urethra, the tube that allows urine and semen to exit the body. Muse therapy is based on the finding that the urethra can absorb certain medications into the surrounding erectile tissues, thereby creating an erection. Muse may have fewer side effects than oral medications because it is used locally. Side effects may include pain in the penis, testicle, or groin; minor bleeding or spotting from the penis; dizziness; swelling (especially of the veins in the legs); and rapid heartbeat.

Vacuum erection device (VED) is a clear plastic cylinder that is placed over the penis. The man then uses a pump to draw out the air, creating a vacuum. This negative pressure draws blood into the penis. A constrictive band may be placed at the base of the penis to prevent a backflow of blood and prolong the erection. A main advantage of this method is that it doesn't require an intact nervous connection. This technique has also been useful in preventing any shortening of the penis, which can occur post-therapy, especially when begun soon after prostatectomy.

Because prostate cancer is sensitive to the presence of male sex hormones, many men with clinically localized, intermediate to high-risk prostate cancer will also receive a six-month to three-year course of androgen deprivation therapy (ADT). Decreased levels of testosterone can lead to body changes in men, including gynecomastia (growth of breast tissue), decrease in the size of the penis and testicles, and thinning of body hair.

--------------- MY JOURNEY ---------------

I don't know which was worse: the side effects of radiation, or not being able to get it up for my girlfriend. All I can say is, thank God when the treatment ended and I was able to slowly return to my normal self. I am forever grateful to my sweetheart for sticking with me. I've heard many stories of relationships cracking up because the man couldn't perform. Ladies, give us a break, okay? This is the last thing we want to happen! First, we want to live, and then we're ready to do just about anything to keep you happy. So hang in there. We need you now more than ever.

Jeff (Denver, Colorado)

Infertility

Many cancer treatments and some types of cancer can cause fertility-related side effects. Radiation therapy to the pelvic area (anus, bladder, penis, or prostate), chemotherapy, and surgery for penile, rectal, prostate, and testicular cancers are all factors that can affect fertility.

Men with testicular cancer are particularly affected by questions of fertility. Unlike prostate cancer, which tends to strike older men, testicular cancer is typically found in young men in the prime of their reproductive years.

Infertility in men with testicular cancer can occur for several reasons. Preexisting conditions, such as cryptorchidism and testicular atrophy, both of which can lead to impaired sperm production, also put men at increased risk for testicular cancer. In addition, low sperm counts have been found in about a third of men at the time of the diagnosis. Low sperm mobility has been found in about half of those in pretreatment. At this time, it is not known whether this is related to changes caused by the tumor itself or from any preexisting medical conditions.

Treatment for testicular cancer can also cause fertility issues. Removal of one of the testes (orchiectomy) is the most common first step in testicular cancer treatment. Having one testicle—no matter what the cause—by no means rules out fertility; however, it may be more difficult due to lower sperm counts.

Radiation therapy and chemotherapy can also affect sperm production. Radiation to the pelvis can damage sperm and impair their function. It is also advised that men who have had pelvic radiation therapy avoid pregnancy in their partners for several weeks after treatment. Chemotherapy, particularly with cisplatin, etoposide, and bleomycin (BEP), can also cause a drop in spermatogenesis (the production of sperm), which reaches its low point at around a year after treatment. However, three-quarters of men will recover sperm counts within three years.

Even men with low sperm counts can father children, especially with a procedure called intracytoplasmic sperm injection, in which a single sperm is injected into an egg.

Take It to the Bank: Fertility Preservation in Men

Given the unwelcome effects on fertility from surgery, radiation therapy, and chemotherapy, it is vital to inform men *prior* to beginning treatment of their options for fertility preservation.

If becoming a parent is important to you, talk with your physician *before* beginning any treatment. In 2006, the American Society of Clinical Oncology (ASCO) published guidelines recommending that oncologists discuss with all patients of reproductive age the possibility of treatment-related infertility, as well as options for preserving fertility, and provide them with referrals to reproductive specialists.

The simplest strategy is to collect semen for cryostorage, otherwise known as sperm banking. The sample is typically collected by masturbation. Although this may seem like an embarrassing or uncomfortable thing to do, most centers offer private, comfortable places for sample collection. With proper instruction, it is possible to collect a sample at home, but since the specimen must be kept at body temperature, it must be brought to the lab within forty-five to sixty minutes after collection. Lubricants, including spit or saliva, should be avoided as they can contaminate the sample. If possible, multiple specimen donations are recommended, with at least a few days between donations.

A sample can be collected using a condom; however, a special condom must be used, as most commercially available condoms contain a spermicide, which kills sperm.

Sperm banks usually "wash" the sperm sample to extract sperm from the rest of the material in the semen. A cryoprotectant semen extender is added if the sperm is to be placed in frozen storage. One sample can produce anywhere from one to twenty vials or straws, depending on the quantity of the ejaculate and whether the sample is washed or unwashed. Unwashed samples are used for intracervical insemination (ICI) treatments, while washed samples are used in intrauterine insemination (IUI) and for in vitro fertilization (IVF) procedures.

Sperm are a little tricky to freeze because of their water content. Slow freezing could form ice crystals, which could damage the sperm when thawed. In a newer process called vitrification, sperm is placed in a bath with a chemical called cryoprotectant (think of it like anti-freeze), along with sucrose. This helps draw out some of the water and replaces it with the cryoprotectant. The sperm is then instantly frozen using liquid nitrogen at −196 degrees.

After cryopreservation, semen can be used successfully for an indefinite period. For human sperm, the longest reported successful storage is twenty-two years.

Costs for sperm banking can run from $1,000 on up for the analysis and freezing, plus $300 to $500 per year for storage. However, costs vary greatly from center to center, so it is important to compare costs at clinics in your area. Some even offer less expensive prepaid plans. Check with your insurance company to see if any of these costs are covered. Some programs offer financial assistance for those who may need additional aid.[33]

A few other procedures have been developed for men for whom routine sperm banking is not feasible. Testicular sperm extraction (TESE) is the process of removing a small portion of tissue from the testicle under local anesthesia and extracting the few viable sperm cells present in that tissue. These viable sperm can then be used for intracytoplasmic sperm injection (ICSI). Check with your medical team for more detailed information.

───────────────── **MY JOURNEY** ─────────────────

I never thought I'd be banking sperm. I was way too young, and as an amateur athlete, I thought I was too fit to get sick like that. After I was diagnosed with testicular cancer, I ended up at one of those clinics feeling like a high school kid doing something wrong behind the barn or something. It was extremely awkward, but now, with two

───────────────────

33. *www.livestrong.org/we-can-help/fertility-services/*

kids running around our house, I am beyond happy that I got over my embarrassment and took care of business. My kids are the best things that ever happened to me, next to living long enough to raise them.

Norris (Casper, Wyoming)

Questions for Your Healthcare Team
About Sexuality and Fertility

Many boys learned in the Boy Scouts that preparation is everything, so why not apply those same principles regarding visiting your doctors? Consider adding these questions to your list:

- What problems might I have during or after treatment, and how long might these last?
- Will any of these problems be permanent?
- How can these problems be treated or managed?
- Could you give me the name of a specialist I can talk with to learn more?
- What precautions do I need to take during treatment?
- Do I need to use a condom?
- Can you recommend a support group for men?
- Will the treatment make me infertile (unable to have children in the future)?
- What are all of my options if I would like to have children in the future?
- Could you refer me to a fertility specialist where I can learn more?
- After treatment, how long should I use some method of birth control?

Urinary Problems

After prostate cancer treatment, men usually face two main types of urinary problems: incontinence and irritative voiding. Urinary incontinence can range from mild leakage of urine to complete loss of bladder control. Irritative voiding symptoms include increased frequency of urination, urinary urgency (feeling like you have to go right away), and pain with urination. Both of these problems are due to damage to the nerves and muscles responsible for urinary control, and any cancer treatment can cause either.

According to the Prostate Cancer Foundation, on average about "25 percent of men report frequent leakage or no control and a need to use absorbent pads at six months after treatment; by three years, fewer than 10 percent report using pads at all."[34]

Irritative urinary symptoms are believed to occur secondary to inflammation of the bladder neck/urethra. Drugs that improve urinary flow can relieve symptoms. Alpha-blockers, such as tamsulosin (Flomax) and terazosin (Hytrin), are typically started in all men following radiation therapy. They are used for at least a few weeks and may be gradually withdrawn as the patient's symptoms improve. Some men may need to be treated for longer periods of time. Anticholinergic medications, like tolterodine (Detrol) or solifenacin (Vesicare), can also help treat irritative bladder symptoms.

Incontinence is also treatable, though no single treatment works for everyone. Your treatment will depend on the type and severity of your problem, lifestyle, and preferences, starting with the simpler treatment options. For example, absorbent pads and pants can be worn inside your underwear, or instead of underwear. They soak up any leaks and are usually very discreet, so people won't know you're wearing them.

---

34. *http://www.pcf.org/site/c.leJRIROrEpH/b.5814053/k.1572/Urinary_Dysfunction.htm*

For some men, avoiding incontinence is as simple as limiting fluids at certain times of the day, or planning regular trips to the bathroom—a therapy called timed voiding or bladder training. As you gain control, you can extend the time between trips.

Kegel exercises are also used for bladder training to strengthen the pelvic muscles, which help hold urine in the bladder. Extensive studies have not yet conclusively shown that Kegel exercises are effective in reducing incontinence in men, but many clinicians find them to be an important element of therapy.

--------------------------------- MY JOURNEY ---------------------------------

I had my prostate removed five years ago because of cancer. I had bladder control problems for the first three months. But with proper exercise I was able to control my bladder. As far as my sex life was concerned, the first year sucked. But as time went by I am now about 85 percent back to normal. Of course, an understanding partner sure helps. So you guys, hang on. It gets better as time goes by.

Marco (Santa Monica, California)

Kegel 101

The first step in Kegel exercises is to find the right muscles. Imagine that you are trying to stop yourself from passing gas. Squeeze the muscles you would use. If you sense a pulling feeling, those are the right muscles for pelvic exercises.

Do not squeeze other muscles at the same time or hold your breath. Also, be careful not to tighten your stomach, leg, or buttock muscles. Squeezing the wrong muscles can put more pressure on your bladder control muscles. Squeeze just the pelvic muscles. Pull them in and hold for a count of three. Then relax for a count of three. Repeat, but do not overdo it. Work up to three sets of ten repeats. Start doing your pelvic muscle exercises lying down. This position is the easiest for doing Kegel exercises because the muscles do not work against gravity. When your muscles get stronger, do your exercises while sitting or standing. Working against gravity is like adding more weight.

Be patient. Do not give up. It takes just five minutes three times a day. Your bladder control may not improve for three to six weeks, although most people notice an improvement after a few weeks.

Harry Belafonte: Grace Under Pressure

Singer, songwriter, actor, and social activist Harry Belafonte isn't afraid of talking about prostate cancer and its conversational taboos—incontinence and impotence.

The "King of Calypso" was diagnosed in 1996 after blood work done during routine checkups showed a rising PSA level. He underwent a prostatectomy and, like many men, had urinary incontinence after the procedure.

He told 500 guests at a benefit for the Hoag Cancer Center in Newport Beach in 1997 that he had problems with incontinence. "But, because I was tenacious about doing the [curative] exercises, after one year it no longer existed."[35]

And, yes, he and his wife still enjoy a level of physical affection that "unifies our lives."

Belafonte took on prostate cancer as another of his noble causes, wanting to raise awareness about the disease and its complications. As he told Penn Medicine's *Oncolink*, "Even in the world of incontinence, you can always do things to improve it. There are exercises that really work. Plus, this is a function of age, too. As men and women get older many of them have incontinence anyway. When you measure the

---

35. http://articles.latimes.com/1997-04-21/news/ls-50829_1_prostate-cancer

level of discomfort that incontinence adds to your life and weigh that against survival and life itself, it seems too insignificant."[36]

Surgical Treatments

Surgical treatments can help men with incontinence resulting from nerve-damaging treatments, such as radiation therapy or radical prostatectomy.

Some men may eliminate urine leakage with an artificial sphincter, an implanted device that keeps the urethra closed until you are ready to urinate. This device can help people who have incontinence because of weak sphincter muscles or because of nerve damage that interferes with sphincter muscle function. It does not solve incontinence caused by uncontrolled bladder contractions.

Surgery to place the artificial sphincter requires general or spinal anesthesia. The device has three parts: a cuff that fits around the urethra, a small balloon reservoir placed in the abdomen, and a pump placed in the scrotum. The cuff is filled with liquid that makes it fit tightly around the urethra to prevent urine from leaking. When it is time to urinate, you squeeze the pump with your fingers to deflate the cuff so that the liquid moves to the balloon reservoir and urine can flow through the urethra. When your bladder is empty, the cuff automatically refills in the next two to five minutes to keep the urethra tightly closed.

Another option is the male sling. In this procedure, the surgeon creates a support for the urethra by wrapping a strip of material around the urethra and attaching the ends of the strip to the pelvic bone. The sling keeps constant pressure on the urethra so that it does not open until the patient consciously releases the urine.

---

36. *http://www.oncolink.org/types/article.cfm?c=1517&id=9492*

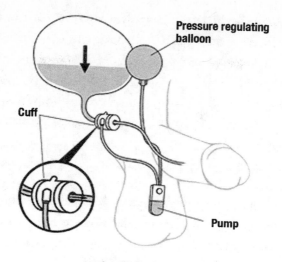

Artificial Sphincter
Source: National Institute of Diabetes and Digestive and Kidney Diseases

---

MY JOURNEY

It felt like I was peeing or leaking or spilling fluid wherever I went, twenty-four hours a day. I couldn't stop it. I was a big, overgrown baby trucking around town in my diapers. Luckily, nobody knew, except for my wife, and she teased me like crazy. I guess it was her way of coping with a very uncomfortable situation. I can't blame her. But at least I changed myself!

Mike (Charlotte, North Carolina)

Two Cancers in One Lifetime?

As the population of cancer survivors continues to grow, with over 14.5 million in the United States in 2014 and a projected increase by 2 percent each year, there is a great need to better understand the long-term health of this population. Nearly one in five cancers diagnosed today occurs in an individual with a previous diagnosis of cancer, and these "second cancers" are a leading cause of morbidity and mortality among cancer survivors. The National Cancer Institute's Surveillance, Epidemiology, and End Results (SEER) program documents that survivors have a 14 percent higher risk of developing a second cancer than would be expected in the general population.

Before proceeding, here are a few definitions to clarify the timeline:

- *Primary cancer* is a term used to describe the original (first) tumor in the body. Cancer cells from a primary cancer may spread to other parts of the body and form new or metastatic tumors. These secondary tumors are the same type of cancer as the primary cancer.
- *A second cancer* refers to a completely new primary cancer in a person with a history of cancer.
- *Field cancerization* is a term that describes the phenomenon where a cancer patient later gets a second cancer either in the same organ or an organ located near the first cancer. Scientists postulate that the increased risk for this second cancer is that the surrounding tissues were exposed to the same cancer-causing agents as the first cancer. Examples of field cancerization include colorectal, breast, lung, bladder, and head and neck cancers.

Pete Postlethwaite: Actor, Not Cancer Victim

Although you may not recognize his name, you will certainly recognize his distinctive face from such movies as *The Usual Suspects*, *The Town*, and *Inception*. British actor Pete Postlethwaite was nominated for an Oscar for his role in *In the Name of the Father*. Steven Spielberg, who worked with Postlethwaite in *Jurassic Park, The Lost World,* and *Amistad,* called him "probably the best actor in the world today."

Postlethwaite had been successfully treated for testicular cancer in 1990. Although he had one testicle removed, he fathered a daughter, Lily, in 1996.

In March 2009, Postlethwaite went to his doctor, complaining of weight loss and fatigue. Tests revealed a large malignant tumor on one of his kidneys. He underwent surgery to have the kidney removed then returned to work, performing in *Clash of the Titans, The Town,* and *Inception.* Pete underwent several grueling rounds of chemotherapy but tried to remain hopeful. As he wrote in his autobiography, *A Spectacle of Dust,* "Weak or not, I was brutal about giving my best. Actor, not cancer victim: that was my mantra."

Although Postlethwaite's doctor saw some initial improvement just before his final round of chemotherapy, when Pete later visited his doctor, he did not receive good news. His tumor was still growing and an additional round of chemotherapy would not defeat it, as it was inoperable.

Pete Postlethwaite died on January 2, 2011, at the age of sixty-four.

Two Too Many

Why are cancer survivors at higher risk of a second cancer? The answer is probably a combination of multiple factors, including:

- *Lifestyle and environmental factors:* Some cancers are caused by known cancer-producing agents, such as smoking, alcohol, and HPV infection. Smokers can get cancer of the larynx (voice box) but are also at risk of getting lung or esophageal cancer. HPV infections can cause cervical infection as well as head and neck cancer.

- *Genetic susceptibility:* As discussed in Chapter 3, some families pass down abnormal genetic changes, increasing the risk for cancer. The BRCA1 and BRCA2 genes put women (and men) at increased risk for breast cancer as well as ovarian cancer.

  Families with Lynch syndrome (hereditary non-polyposis colorectal cancer syndrome) have an increased risk for cancers of the stomach, small intestine, liver, gallbladder ducts, upper urinary tract, brain, and skin (See Chapter 3.)

Previous cancer treatments, including the following, can contribute to secondary cancers:

Radiation Therapy

Going back to the study of survivors of the atomic bomb blasts in Japan, exposure to radiation has been known for many years to be a potential cause of cancer. Workers exposed to radiation in their jobs and cancer patients who have received radiotherapy are also at higher risk of cancer caused by their exposure.

Many kinds of blood cancers as well as solid tumors can be linked to previous radiation therapy. Several kinds of leukemia, including acute myelogenous leukemia (AML), chronic myelogenous leukemia (CML), and acute lymphoblastic leukemia (ALL), as well as a bone marrow cancer called myelodysplastic syndrome (see the story of Robin Roberts in this chapter) can all be caused by previous radiation exposure. The increase in risk is dependent on the amount of radiation the bone marrow received during treatment. These cancers tend to occur within a few years after radiation therapy, typically within five to nine years after exposure.

Solid tumors, which are caused by radiation therapy, tend to occur much later, perhaps even ten to fifteen years or more after exposure. The risk is dependent on the dose of radiation, the patient's age at the time of treatment (higher risk in younger patients), and the area where the radiation was given. Some organs, such as breast and thyroid, are more sensitive to the effects than others.

Chemotherapy

This has also been linked to second cancers. The most common cancers linked to chemotherapy are myelodysplastic syndrome (MDS) and AML. Some patients develop MDS, which later turns into AML. The risk of these cancers is higher with chemotherapy than with radiation therapy.

Alkylating agents, such as mechlorethamine, chlorambucil, cyclophosphamide (Cytoxan), melphalan, lomustine (CCNU), carmustine (BCNU), and busulfan are all known to cause leukemia and MDS. Higher drug dose and dose intensity as well as longer therapy duration increase the risk of leukemia. The risk is greatest beginning two years after treatment and reaches its peak five to ten years after exposure.

Other chemotherapeutic drugs known to cause leukemia include cisplatin and carboplatin, as well as a class of drugs called topoisomerase II inhibitors. They work by stopping cancer cells from being able to repair DNA. One subset of topoisomerase II inhibitors called anthracyclines is less likely to cause leukemia. However, as previously mentioned, they can have toxic effects on the heart.

Stem Cell Transplant

This is a method of giving chemotherapy and then replacing blood-forming cells destroyed by the treatment. Stem cells (immature blood cells) are removed from the blood or bone marrow of a donor and frozen for storage. Patients then receive high doses of chemotherapy/ radiation therapy. Upon completion, the stored stem cells are thawed and placed in the patient through an infusion. These reinfused stem cells grow into (and restore) the body's blood cells.

Any type of stem cell transplant puts a patient at increased risk of second cancer because of the chemo and radiation therapy received. In addition, patients who receive stem cells from a donor will need to be on drugs to suppress their immune system to prevent rejection of the donor's stem cells. As some cells of the immune system recognize cancer cells as abnormal and kill them, immune suppressive drugs can decrease this ability.

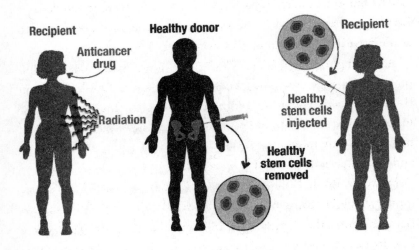

Allogeneic Stem Cell Transplant

The Case of Robin Roberts and the Need for Minority Donors

Good Morning America anchor Robin Roberts was diagnosed with cancer in 2007. She underwent surgery, chemotherapy, and six weeks of radiation therapy. Despite this, she returned to the anchor desk only a couple of weeks later, wearing a wig because she "didn't want to distract viewers from the news."

In 2012, Roberts was diagnosed with MDS, a group of diseases in which the bone marrow does not make enough healthy blood cells, and researchers think that it may have been the result of radiation or chemotherapy Roberts had previously received.

She needed a stem cell transplant, which is a method of giving chemotherapy and replacing blood-forming cells destroyed by the treatment. Her sister became her donor, and five months later, Robin Roberts triumphantly returned to *Good Morning America*.

In a show of support, her colleagues promoted bone marrow donation by sponsoring a registry drive. *GMA*'s George Stephanopoulos and Lara Spencer as well as ABC News president Ben Sherwood showed up at the drive and had their cheeks swabbed to join the registry.

According to Jeffrey Chell, CEO of Be The Match,[37] over 44,000 people have registered with the National Marrow Donor Program (NMDR) since Roberts announced her diagnosis. This is over 20,000 more than the registry would normally receive in that period! It is estimated that sixty to seventy of these new donors will be a good match and have their marrow used in a transplant.

However, Robin Robert's bone marrow transplant also highlights a more pressing problem, which is an acute shortage of minority donors. Because of this, the chance of finding a match on the national registry is as low as 76 percent for African Americans and other minorities, compared with 97 percent for Caucasians.

Of the over 9 million potential donors in the Be The Match registry, Caucasians constitute nearly three-quarters of the donors. Hispanics are at 10 percent, and Asians and African Americans are at 7 percent each. As HLA typing tends to be closest within racial groups, this can make finding a suitable donor a difficult proposition.

In multiracial populations, the problem is even more acute. According to the 2010 census, the multiracial population among American children has increased almost 50 percent since 2000. This makes it the fastest growing youth group in the country.

---

37. *https://bethematch.org/*

Programs have been established to increase awareness in communities, with a special emphasis on African Americans, American Indian–Alaskan Natives, Asian-Pacific Islanders, and Hispanics. One of these is the National MOTTEP[38] (National Minority Organ and Tissue Transplant Education Program), whose mission is to educate ethnic minority Americans about the need for organ, tissue, and blood donations. MOTTEP simultaneously educates communities about the diseases and behaviors that lead to the need for transplantation.

MY JOURNEY

I've met several men in my prostate cancer support group who are still dealing with pee problems and having trouble getting it up and dealing with life, in general. Even after the actual cancer is gone, you got a lot to still deal with, and the physical things are just one piece of the puzzle. But there are plenty of men out there going through the same crap you are, and they're just glad to be alive and figure something else besides cancer will eventually kill 'em, so why make such a fuss? I suggest you seek them out and don't be so stubborn about fixing it all yourself. That ain't gonna happen, most likely, because who can do that all by himself?

Sonny (Chicago, Illinois)

Survivorship and Quality of Life

With more long-term cancer survivors on record in the United States than ever before, it is imperative that we enhance our understanding of the dynamics of their survivorship and how it affects the

---

38. *http://www.mottep.org/*

whole person, not just physical symptoms and health, but an overall quality of life.

According to a 1997 review article in *Oncology* by Betty R. Ferrell, PhD, RN, and Karen Hassey Dow, PhD, RN, "Quality of life (QOL) issues have become a vital area of concern to cancer survivors, their families, and care providers," and "future advances in cancer treatment will further heighten the importance of survivorship issues in comprehensive cancer care."

The *European Journal of Cancer* urged in 2005 that because of the growing numbers of long-term breast cancer survivors, specific treatments need to be adapted in order to accommodate and support this trend. Their research showed that women who survived longer after a diagnosis of breast cancer reported a better overall quality of life and better psychological and social well-being than women with fewer years of survival.

Since then, studies of breast cancer patients have found that when psychosocial care is added to a patient's general treatment, her short- *and* long-term quality of life may be significantly improved, especially compared with women who did not receive this intervention.

On another front, studies prove that psychosocial care not only improves a patient's health, it also reduces healthcare billings by 24 percent in women who attended psychosocial intervention projects compared with women who did not.[39]

These issues are not new and many of the same lessons can be applied to men. They began to come to the forefront beginning in 1990 when the National Cancer Institute (NCI) began using QOL measures to compare treatments, as well as having them serve as markers for treatment trials, general assessors of rehabilitation needs, and predictors of future responses to a variety of treatments. The NCI

---

39. *https://www.researchgate.net/publication/7540830*

continues to expand its use of QOL controls in clinical trials, research, and outcome studies, with special emphasis to assess QOL in culturally diverse populations.

A growing number of cancer centers throughout the country are increasing their resources to support and treat the long-term implications of cancer treatment, including the consequences men face when dealing with gender-specific cancers.

In the next chapter, we will explore a wide range of conventional and complementary treatments that address many of these issues.

KEY POINTS TO REMEMBER

✓ One in four people with cancer reports memory and attention problems after chemotherapy. This is commonly referred to as chemo brain.

✓ Dealing with cancer can lead to serious depression, severe emotional distress, fear of recurrence, and interference with sleep.

✓ Radiation therapy can lead to GI symptoms, such as ulcers, proctitis, and enteritis.

✓ Chemotherapy (especially bleomycin and cisplatin) used to treat testicular cancer can cause temporary or permanent lung problems.

✓ Patients with preexisting medical conditions may be at higher risk of cardiotoxic effects from chemotherapy/radiation therapy.

✓ All patients undergoing chemotherapy should have a pretreatment heart evaluation.

✓ Sexual dysfunction (impotence) is a frequent complication of men's cancer treatments.

✓ Penile rehabilitation programs can help men with erectile dysfunction recover function.

✓ Infertility is an important issue for men undergoing cancer treatment.

✓ Fertility preservation options should be discussed before any treatment begins.

✓ Urinary problems, both incontinence and irritative symptoms, are common after prostate cancer treatment. Fortunately, most improve over time.

✓ Any patient who has had cancer has an increased risk of having a second cancer.

WHAT CANCER CANNOT DO

Cancer is so limited . . .
It cannot cripple love.
It cannot shatter hope.
It cannot corrode faith.
It cannot eat away peace.
It cannot destroy confidence.
It cannot kill friendship.
It cannot shut out memories.

It cannot silence courage.

9

CONVENTIONAL AND COMPLEMENTARY WISDOM: Managing the Side Effects of Cancer Treatments

When you come to the end of your rope,
tie a knot and hang on.

—Franklin D. Roosevelt

What's New?

I n Chapters 7 and 8, we discussed many of the residual issues affecting men during a cancer journey. Now we'd like to help you manage as many of those short- and long-term side effects as possible.

When someone is diagnosed with cancer, he wants to do everything possible to combat the disease, as well as manage its symptoms and cope with any consequences of treatment. Many turn to complementary health options, including natural products—such as herbs and dietary supplements, medical marijuana—and mind and body practices, including acupuncture, massage, and yoga, as well as writing and an assortment of art therapy.

This introductory overview of these approaches is based on collaboration between the U.S. National Center for Complementary and Integrative Health (NCCIH) and the U.S. National Cancer Institute (NCI). These options have been studied for cancer prevention, cancer treatment, or symptom management. We'll include what the science says about their effectiveness as well as any concerns about their safety.

Anemia

This condition refers to a lower than normal red blood cell count, which most often leads to fatigue along with pale skin in some people. Here's what we recommend:

Save your energy. Don't be afraid to ask for help. Figure out your most important tasks for the day, and when people offer to help, let them. They can take you to the doctor, empty the dishwasher, make meals, or do other things you are too tired to do.

Balance rest with activity. Take short naps during the day, but keep in mind that too much bed rest can make you feel weak. You may feel better if you take short walks or exercise a little every day. Even five minutes of activity here and there can do wonders.

Eat and drink well. You may need to eat foods that are high in protein or iron. Your doctor, nurse, or a registered dietitian can help decide what foods are best for you. The familiar adage "You are what you eat" could not be more accurate when it comes to treating and preventing disease—of *any* kind.

NOTE to PATIENT:
If you have cancer, seek nutritional counseling.

Loss of Appetite

Take these steps to ensure that you are getting the nutrition you need to stay strong during and after treatment:

Drink plenty of liquids. Losing fluid can lead to dehydration, a dangerous condition. You may become weak or dizzy and have dark yellow urine if you are not drinking enough liquids.

Choose healthy and high-nutrient foods. Eat a little, even if you are not hungry. Have five or six small meals throughout the day instead of three large meals. Try to eat nutrient-dense foods that are high in protein and calories. Keep a supply of tasty, quality protein bars on hand.

Stay active. Movement will actually increase your appetite. Even taking a short walk each day can help. Taking one of those protein bars with you when you're out—along with a bottle of water—will come in handy.

Bleeding and Bruising

Take these steps if you are at increased risk of bleeding and bruising:

Avoid certain medicines. Many over-the-counter medicines contain aspirin or ibuprofen, which can increase your risk of bleeding. When in doubt, check the label. You may also be advised to limit or avoid alcohol if your platelet count is low.

Take extra care to prevent bleeding. Brush your teeth gently, with a very soft toothbrush. Wear shoes, even when you are inside. Be extra careful when using sharp objects. Use an electric shaver instead of a razor. Use lotion and a lip balm to prevent dry, chapped skin and lips.

Tell your doctor or nurse if you are constipated or notice bleeding from your rectum. If you do start to bleed, press down firmly on the area with a clean cloth. Keep pressing until the bleeding stops. If you bruise, put ice on the area.

MY JOURNEY

Cancer has caused me to depend on other people in ways I never previously imagined. I was always a self-sufficient person and didn't even know how to ask for help. So when I became perpetually tired during treatment, I had to suck it up and basically beg. Once I did, I couldn't stop. And the remarkable thing is, I think my friends actually *liked* helping me!

Shanaya (St. Louis, Missouri)

Constipation

Follow these tips to prevent or treat constipation:

Eat high-fiber foods. Adding bran to food, such as cereals or smoothies, is an easy way to get more fiber in your diet.

Drink plenty of liquids. Most people need to drink at least eight cups of liquid each day. You may require more based on your treatment, medications you are taking, or other health factors. Drinking warm or hot liquids may also help.

Try to be active every day. Most people can do light exercise, even in a bed or chair. Other people choose to walk or ride an exercise bike for fifteen to thirty minutes each day.

Use medicines and treatments prescribed by your doctor. Some over-the-counter products may lead to bleeding, infection, or other harmful side effects.

Diarrhea

Following are ideas to prevent complications from diarrhea:

Drink plenty of fluid each day. Diarrhea causes the body to lose fluids rapidly, and dehydration could develop if you're not drinking enough water.

Eat small meals. This is easier on your stomach and digestive system. For most people, foods high in potassium and sodium (minerals lost when you have diarrhea) are good choices.

Check with your doctor or nurse before taking medicine. Your doctor will prescribe the correct diarrhea medicine for you.

Keep your anal area clean and dry. Use warm water and wipes to stay clean. It may help to take warm, shallow baths (sitz baths).

Fatigue

This is a common side effect of many cancer treatments, including chemotherapy, radiation therapy, biological therapy, bone marrow transplant, and surgery. Co-conditions such as anemia, as well as pain, medications, and emotions can also cause or worsen fatigue.

People often describe cancer-related fatigue as feeling extremely tired, weak, heavy, run down, and having no energy. Resting does not always help with cancer-related fatigue. This is one of the most difficult side effects to cope with for many people.

Try some of these solutions:

Make a plan that balances rest and activity. Choose relaxing activities. For example, listen to music, write, read, meditate, practice guided imagery, or spend time with people you enjoy. Any of these can preserve energy and lower stress. You doctor may also advise light exercise to give you more energy and help you feel better. If you do get tired, take short naps (less than an hour) during the day. Too much sleep during the day can make it difficult to sleep enough at night.

Eat and drink well. Foods high in protein and calories will help you maintain your strength. Eat several small meals throughout the day instead of three big meals. Stay well hydrated. Limit your intake of caffeine and alcohol.

Meet with a specialist. It may help to meet with a counselor, psychologist, or psychiatrist. These experts help people to cope with difficult thoughts and feelings. Lowering stress may give you more energy. Since uncontrolled pain can also be major source of fatigue, it may help to meet with a pain or palliative care specialist.

> **NOTE to PATIENT:**
> Palliative care is not specifically end-of-life care.
> It offers you a plan to manage pain and
> can be quite temporary.

MY JOURNEY

I was in denial when I first got diagnosed, and it wasn't until my Gleason score shot up that I really took it seriously. Meanwhile, my wife and I took a great trip together, and knowing my marriage was in a good place I felt that I could start what was probably going to be some brutal treatment. Well, the radiation beat me up real good, and I am still struggling mightily a year later. In fact, I don't know my prognosis right now, and my doctors seem noncommittal. But my wife loves me. I take it one day at a time, knowing full well now that

I may not have many left. But I have love, and so far that is carrying me pretty well.

Rudolf (Berlin, Connecticut)

Hair Loss

For those receiving chemo or radiation therapy, hair can fall out slowly or seemingly overnight depending on a number of factors. But no matter how it happens, there are ways to manage it:

Treat your hair gently. You may choose a hairbrush with soft bristles or a wide-tooth comb. Do not use hair dryers, irons, or products such as gels or clips that may hurt your scalp. Wash your hair less often and with a mild shampoo. Be very gentle. Pat it dry with a soft towel.

Shorten or shave? Some people choose to cut their hair short to make it easier to deal with when it starts to fall out. Others choose to shave their heads. If you choose to shave your head, use an electric shaver so you won't cut yourself. If you plan to buy a wig, get one while you still have hair so you can match it to your current or natural color.

Protect and care for your scalp. Use sunscreen or wear a hat when you are outside. Choose something you enjoy that is comfortable and keeps your head warm. If your scalp itches or feels tender, lotions and conditioners (without harsh chemicals) can help it feel better.

Anger, depression, and embarrassment are all common reactions to hair loss. It can help to share these feelings with someone who understands. Some people find it helpful to write down their feelings/ talk with other people who have lost their hair during cancer treatment.

Will It Grow Back?

Yes. After chemotherapy treatment has ended, hair often grows back in two to three months. It will be very fine when it starts growing again. Sometimes, it can be curlier or straighter—or even a different color or shade—than it was prior to loss. Eventually, it may return to how it was before treatment.

After radiation therapy has ended, hair usually grows back within three to six months. If you received a very high dose of radiation, your hair may grow back thinner or not at all on the part of your body that received radiation.

In any case, no matter what type of treatment you received, be gentle with your hair when it begins growing back. Avoid too much brushing, curling, and blow-drying. You may not want to wash your hair as frequently, either, until it feels stronger. Avoid shampoos and conditioners with harsh chemicals, and definitely stay away from coloring your hair unless you are 100 percent sure the dye is chemical-free and safe for use.

From now on, mild, organic products are your best option.

—————————— **MY JOURNEY** ——————————

Before I was diagnosed, I never paid attention to what I ate or what shampoo I used or how many bottles I recycled. But that's all changed now, and I think it will stick. When I eat right, with actual fresh food and no garbage, I feel way better. I cut out all the poison around me too, in things like cleansers and soaps and all the stuff we never realize is hurting us until it might be too late. Maybe I got cancer from all this terrible stuff I've been breathing in and putting on my skin for all these years. So I'm telling everybody to go organic and save yourself while you save the planet. That's right. I'm a stubborn old-fashioned man, and I've been converted!

David (Little Rock, Arkansas)

Preventing Infection

When it comes to hygiene, common sense is a good place to begin, but there are a few more factors to keep in mind during treatment:

Wash your hands often and well. Use soap and warm water, especially before eating. Have people around you wash their hands, too.

Stay extra clean. If you have a catheter, keep the area around it clean and dry. Brush your teeth well, and check your mouth each day for sores or other signs of infection. If you get a scrape or cut, clean it well. Let your doctor or nurse know if your bottom is sore or bleeds, as this can increase your risk of infection.

Avoid human germs. Stay away from people who are sick or have a cold. Avoid crowds and people who have just had a live vaccine, such as for chicken pox, polio, or measles. As people in some parts of Asia often do when they are sick while out and about, consider wearing a breathable facemask if you're traveling in a crowded environment, like a subway or train.

Monitor your food hygiene. Follow food safety guidelines by making sure that the meat, fish, and eggs you eat are well-cooked. Keep hot foods hot and cold foods cold. You may be advised to eat only fruits and vegetables that can be peeled, or to wash all raw fruits and vegetables very well. In fact, it's always wise to thoroughly wash any type of raw food.

—————————— **MY JOURNEY** ——————————

It was terribly hot when I first underwent radiation therapy. I had a very abstract painting that reminded me of Salvador Dali drawn on my chest to remind everyone where I was supposed to get cooked, and they told me to keep the area dry for the next two months. That was definitely a challenge—one that I felt like I was failing almost every

time I took a shower. I wasn't supposed to wear deodorant either, at
least not the kind one usually finds in the average pharmacy. Finally,
after asking around, I discovered a product made from seaweed and a
bunch of other organic minerals. My doctor balked at first, but eventually relented. In this case, I taught *him* something he didn't already
know, and I made it through the summer a lot more comfortably.

Kris (Jacksonville, Florida)

Lymphedema

These steps may help prevent lymphedema or keep it from getting
worse:

Protect your skin. Use lotion to avoid dry skin, and use sunscreen.
Consider wearing plastic gloves with cotton lining when working in
order to prevent scratches, cuts, or burns. Keep your feet clean and
dry. Keep your nails clean and short to prevent ingrown nails and
infection. Avoid tight shoes and wear your jewelry loose.

Exercise. Work to keep body fluids moving, especially in places
where lymphedema has developed. Start with gentle exercises that
help you move and contract your muscles. Ask your doctor or nurse
or physical therapist about which exercises are best for you.

Manual lymph drainage. See a trained specialist (a certified
lymphedema therapist) to receive a type of therapeutic massage called
manual lymph drainage. Therapeutic massage works best to lower
lymphedema when given early, before symptoms progress.

Memory and Concentration Problems

It's important for you or a family member to tell your healthcare team if you have difficulty remembering things, thinking, or

concentrating. Take these steps to help manage minor memory or concentration problems:

Plan your day. Do things that require the most concentration during the time of day when you feel best. Get extra rest and plenty of sleep at night. If you need rest during the day, short naps of less than one hour are best. Maintain a daily routine as best as you can.

Exercise your body and mind. Exercise can help to decrease stress and keep you feeling more alert. Exercise releases endorphins, also known as "feel-good chemicals," which provide feelings of positivity. Mind-body practices, like meditation, or mental exercises, such as puzzles or games, can also help some people.

Write down—and keep handy—a list of important information. Use a daily planner, recorder, or other electronic device to help you remember important activities. Make a list of important names and phone numbers. Keep it in one place so it's easy to find.

And while you're at it, take time to expand your writing into areas of self-expression, as it's important to get in touch with your feelings during this stressful time.

Mouth and Throat Problems

Cancer treatments are notorious for creating problems in the mouth and throat. Here are a few ideas to help ease those challenges:

For a sore mouth or throat choose foods that are soft, wet, and easy to swallow. Soften dry foods with gravy, sauce, or other liquids. Use a blender to make milkshakes, or blend your food to make it easier to swallow. Ask about pain medicines, such as lozenges or sprays, that numb your mouth and make eating less painful. Avoid food and drinks that can irritate your mouth—crunchy, salty, spicy, or sugary foods—as well as alcoholic drinks. And it should go without saying, do not smoke or use tobacco products.

For a dry mouth drink plenty of liquids because a dry mouth can increase the risk of tooth decay and mouth infections. Keep water handy and sip it often to keep your mouth wet. Suck on ice chips or sugar-free hard candy, eat frozen desserts, or chew sugar-free gum. Use a lip balm. Ask about medicines such as saliva substitutes that can coat, protect, and moisten your mouth and throat. Acupuncture may also help with dry mouth.

Changes to your sense of taste may make foods seem to have no taste at all, or not taste the way they used to. Radiation therapy may cause a change in sweet, sour, bitter, and salty tastes. Chemotherapy drugs may cause an unpleasant chemical or metallic taste in your mouth. If you experience taste changes, try different foods to find ones that taste best to you. Eating cold foods may also help.

Here are some more tips to help you with changing tastes:

- If foods taste bland, marinate them to improve their flavor, or add mild spices.
- If red meat tastes strange, switch to other high-protein foods, such as chicken, eggs, fish, peanut butter, turkey, beans, or dairy products. In fact, limit your red meat intake.
- If foods taste salty, bitter, or acidic, try sweetening them with a bit of honey.
- If foods taste metallic, switch to plastic utensils and nonmetal cooking dishes.
- If you have a bad taste in your mouth, try sugar-free lemon drops, gum, or mints.

MY JOURNEY

Following radiation treatment, I had severe diarrhea, which lasted for several weeks. My doctor told me this might happen and that my rectum might be damaged, but he didn't let on how bad it could really get. I don't know if he didn't want to scare me, but I wish I had been warned a little more because this came on so strong, I thought I would die from my bowels exploding instead of having cancer. I tried experimenting with different diets, and I never figured out what worked best, but eventually my body relaxed and returned to normal, if there even is such a thing.

Frank (Dallas, Texas)

NOTE to PATIENT:
Consult with a cancer-friendly nutritionist!

Nausea and Vomiting

Here are some suggestions that might ease these troublesome side effects:

Take antinausea medicine, which your doctor can prescribe. Most people need to take an antinausea medicine even on days when they feel well. Tell your doctor or nurse if the medicine you're taking doesn't help. Different options may work better for you.

Drink plenty of water and fluids to prevent dehydration. Make a habit of sipping water, fruit juices, ginger ale, tea, and/or sports drinks throughout the day. Be careful to avoid drinks with high sugar content.

Avoid foods that are greasy, fried, sweet, or spicy. This will help, especially if you feel sick after eating them. If the smell of food bothers you while cooking, ask others to make your food. Try cold foods that do not have strong smells, or let food cool down before you eat it.

Eat a small snack before treatment. This can help many people handle those days a little easier. Others avoid eating or drinking right before or after treatment because it makes them feel sick. After treatment, wait at least one hour before you eat or drink.

Learn about complementary medicine practices. For some, acupuncture relieves nausea/vomiting caused by chemotherapy. Deep breathing, guided imagery, hypnosis, and other relaxation techniques (such as listening to music, reading a book, or meditating) may also help. Read more about these options later in this chapter.

Nerves and Senses

If you have experienced nerve changes, you may be advised to take these steps:

Prevent falls. Move rugs so you will not trip on them. Ask for help with this, if needed. Put rails on walls, especially in the bathroom, so you can hold on to them for balance and security. Put bathmats in the shower or tub. Wear sturdy shoes with soft soles. Get up slowly after sitting or lying down, especially if you feel dizzy.

Take extra care in the kitchen and shower. Use potholders in the kitchen to protect your hands from burns. Be careful when handling knives or sharp objects. Ask someone to check the water temperature, to make sure it's not too hot.

Protect your hands and feet. Wear shoes indoors and out. Check your arms, legs, and feet daily for cuts or scratches. If it's cold, wear warm clothes to protect your hands and feet.

Ask for help and slow down. Let people help you with difficult tasks. Slow down and give yourself more time to do things.

Ask about pain medicine and integrative medicine practices. You may be prescribed pain medicine. Other methods, such as acupuncture, massage, physical therapy, and yoga, may also lessen pain. Talk with your healthcare team to learn what is best for you. You can find more about these later in this chapter.

The Pain Game

Here is a guide for you and your healthcare team to prevent, treat, or lessen pain:

Keep track of your pain profile. Each day write about any pain you feel. Specify where it hurts and describe the pain (sharp, burning, shooting, or throbbing). What triggers the pain, and how long does it last? Does it interfere with desired activities, such as eating, sleeping, or working? What makes it feel better—or worse? For example, do ice packs, heating pads, or exercises help? Does pain medicine help? How much do you take and how often? Rate your pain on a scale of one to ten, with ten signifying the most and one the least.

Take pain medicine as prescribed. Don't wait until your pain becomes severe before taking your meds. That can delay relief. Tell your doctor or nurse if the medicine is no longer effective, or if the pain returns before it is time to take the next dose.

Consider meeting with a pain specialist who often works together with a pain or palliative care team and may include a neurologist, surgeon, physiatrist, psychiatrist, psychologist, or pharmacist.

Ask about integrative medicine. Treatments such as acupuncture, biofeedback, hypnosis, massage therapy, and physical therapy may help treat pain.

--- ---------------------------- MY JOURNEY -------------------------

I went into this whole thing pretty blind. I had no idea that my legs would get barbecued from radiation, making me so uncomfortable I could barely walk or sit down. I was able to calm down the situation at home with a lot of ointment, but at work I was screwed. My oncologist gave me some medication to handle the pain, and it eventually became tolerable. I feared becoming addicted to those pills. Luckily, I didn't, and the worst of it finally passed. Now my skin is still uncomfortable sometimes, but it's manageable.

Scott (Hicksville, New York)

Skin Care

Depending on what treatment you are receiving, a host of options are available to protect your skin, prevent infection, and reduce itching.

Use mild soaps that are gentle on your skin. Ask for specific recommendations for lotions and creams, and ask if you should avoid any skin products. For example, you may be advised not use powders or antiperspirants before radiation therapy.

Protect your skin. Lotions or antibiotics may be needed for dry, itchy, infected, or swollen skin. Avoid heating pads, ice packs, or bandages on areas receiving radiation therapy. Shave less often and use an electric razor—or stop shaving—if your skin is sore. When outdoors, wear sunscreen and lip balm, a wide-brimmed hat, and loose fitting pants and long-sleeved shirts.

Prevent or treat dry, itchy skin (pruritus). Avoid products with alcohol or perfume, which can dry or irritate your skin. Take short showers or baths in lukewarm water. Afterward, gently pat yourself dry and immediately put on lotion, while your skin is still slightly damp. Keep your home cool and humid. Eat a healthy diet and drink plenty of fluids to keep your skin moist and healthy. Applying a cool washcloth to the affected area may also help. Consider acupuncture, too.

Prevent or treat minor nail problems. Keep your nails clean and cut short. Wear gloves when you wash dishes, work in the garden, or clean the house.

Sleep Issues

If you're having trouble falling—or staying— asleep, consider these helpful steps:

Tell your doctor about problems that interfere with sleep. Getting treatment to deal with those issues (such as pain or bladder or gastrointestinal problems) may help you sleep better.

Cognitive behavioral therapy (CBT) and relaxation therapy may help. A CBT therapist can help you learn to change negative thoughts and beliefs about sleep into positive ones. Strategies such as muscle relaxation, guided imagery, and self-hypnosis may also help.

Set good bedtime habits. Go to bed only when sleepy in a quiet, dark room in a comfortable bed. If you do not fall asleep, get out of bed then return to bed when you are sleepy. Stop watching television or using other electrical devices a couple of hours before going to bed. Don't drink or eat a lot before bedtime. While it's important to keep active during the day with regular exercise, exercising within a few hours before bedtime may make sleep more difficult.

If other strategies do not work, your doctor may prescribe sleep medicine for a short period. The sleep medicine prescribed will depend on your specific problem (such as trouble falling asleep or trouble staying asleep) as well as other medicines you are taking.

Urinary Symptoms

It's never a bad idea to remind ourselves about staying hydrated, so let's begin with that and add a few other thoughts that contribute to good urinary health.

Drink enough liquid. Urine should be light yellow or clear. Avoid things that can make bladder problems worse, like caffeine, alcohol, spicy foods, and tobacco products.

Lower your chances of getting a urinary tract infection. Go often to the bathroom. Wear cotton underwear and loose-fitting pants. Learn about safe and sanitary practices for catheterization, and take showers instead of baths.

———— MY JOURNEY ————

I was incontinent for six months after my surgery and lived my life from one pad to the next. No matter where I went or what I did, I had to have access to changing them every hour. Even though I had to change my lifestyle in a big way, I'm still glad I went ahead with this treatment.

Luke (Cleveland, Ohio)

Venturing Outside Mainstream Medicine: Complementary, Alternative, and Integrative Options for Managing Side Effects

Once a patient begins investigating other ideas and practices outside the traditional scope of mainstream medicine, he opens up many exciting doors to a variety of healthcare possibilities. Complementary health approaches involve a group of diverse medical and healthcare systems, along with practices and products that originated outside the status quo. These include the use of herbal or other dietary supplements—including medical marijuana—meditation, spinal manipulation, and acupuncture. A worldwide estimate of 33 to 47 percent of people diagnosed with cancer use complementary, alternative, or integrative therapies during their cancer treatment.

Many Americans using these approaches refer to them interchangeably as "alternative" or "complementary," but the terms differ. Complementary refers to a nonmainstream practice being used together with conventional medicine. Alternative refers to a nonmainstream practice replacing conventional medical techniques. Integrative joins conventional and complementary approaches in a coordinated way. This idea has continued to grow within healthcare systems across the United States. Researchers are exploring the potential benefits of integrative health in a variety of situations, including pain management for military personnel and veterans, relief of symptoms in cancer patients and survivors, and programs to promote healthy behavior.

Evaluating complementary healthcare approaches presents challenges. The same careful scientific evaluation that is used to assess conventional therapies should be used to evaluate complementary approaches. Some of these are beginning to find a place in cancer treatment—not as cures, but as additions to treatment plans that may help patients cope with disease symptoms and side effects while improving their overall quality of life.

Although research on the potential value of these integrative programs is in its early stages, some studies have shown promising results. For example, research conducted by the National Center for Complementary and Integrative Health (NCCIH) suggests the following:

- Cancer patients receiving integrative therapies in the hospital have less pain and anxiety.

- Massage therapy may lead to short-term improvements in pain and mood in patients with advanced cancer.
- Yoga may relieve the persistent fatigue that some men experience after breast cancer treatment. It's something you can do in a group or alone, and it is well worth investigating.

A substantial amount of scientific evidence suggests that some complementary health approaches may help to manage some symptoms of cancer and side effects of treatment. For other complementary approaches, the evidence is more limited.

There is no convincing evidence at this time that any complementary health approach is effective in curing cancer or causing it to go into remission.

Read the Fine Print!

Unproven products or practices should not be used to replace or delay conventional medical treatment for cancer. Some complementary approaches can interfere with standard cancer treatments or may present special risks for people who have been diagnosed with cancer. Before using any complementary health approach, speak with your healthcare providers to make sure that all aspects of your care work together. Give them a full picture of what you are currently doing to manage your health and a vision of what you would like to try. This will help to ensure coordinated and safe care.

The Society of Integrated Oncology (SIO) is an international organization "dedicated to encouraging scientific evaluation, dissemination of evidence-based information and appropriate clinical integration of complementary therapies."[40] In 2009, they issued evidence-based clinical practice guidelines for healthcare providers to consider when

---

40. *http://integrativeonc.org/*

incorporating complementary health approaches in the care of cancer patients. The guidelines point out that, when used in addition to conventional therapies, some of these approaches help to control symptoms and enhance patients' well-being.

SIO recommends that physicians should inquire about the use of complementary and alternative therapies as a routine part of initial evaluations of cancer patients.[41] In addition, all patients with cancer should receive guidance about the advantages and limitations of complementary therapies in an open, evidence-based, and patient-centered manner by a qualified professional. Patients should be fully informed of the treatment approach, the nature of the specific therapies, potential risks/benefits, and realistic expectations.

—— MY JOURNEY ——

Since I work in medical research, I know the value of data. But when I got cancer and began a long regimen of surgery and treatment, I knew in my gut that I needed whatever help I could get my hands on—regardless of whether there was data to support it. So I indulged in a variety of herbal supplements, mind-body awareness training, and nutritional counseling. Even though there are very few scientific numbers to support the benefits of any of these supposedly supplemental treatments, I have become convinced, from my own experience and that of others I have observed, that it takes a mixed bag of treatment to cure a patient, and that each of us must determine what feels good and right as we proceed through this crazy adventure.

Carl (Wichita, Kansas)

41. *http://integrativeonc.org/docman-library/uncategorized/65-sio-guidelines-2009/file*

Can Science Support Other Options?

Inside the medical establishment, the debate over complementary, alternative, and integrative treatments continues. Some cancer centers have wholeheartedly embraced a host of these methods and provide them on-site or through off-site partnerships, while other hospitals devoted to cancer care remain skeptical. Regarding insurance companies and what they will pay for, results are mixed and in a steady state of flux. Generally speaking, the jury is still out, but it's clear that trends are moving strongly in the direction of expanding treatment options—not to replace but to support traditional techniques.

So who are we to listen to?

Blending traditional and nontraditional treatments can be a win-win for many people. However, just as patients need to do their due diligence on educating themselves about surgery, chemotherapy, and radiation, they can also gather plenty of information about the pluses and minuses of complementary, alternative, and integrative options.

For example, substantial evidence exists that acupuncture can help cancer patients manage treatment-related nausea and vomiting. However, there isn't enough evidence yet to judge whether acupuncture relieves cancer pain or other symptoms, such as treatment-related hot flashes. Complications from acupuncture are rare, as long as the acupuncturist uses sterile needles and proper procedures. Chemotherapy and radiation therapy weaken the body's immune system, so it's especially important for acupuncturists to follow strict clean-needle procedures when treating cancer patients.

Studies suggest that the herb ginger may help to control nausea related to cancer chemotherapy when used in addition to conventional antinausea medication. Ginger can be ground up and used to make tea and can also be eaten raw, as you may often see it served with sushi as a palate cleanser.

Studies suggest that massage therapy may help to relieve symptoms experienced by people with cancer, such as pain, nausea, anxiety, and depression. You should consult with your healthcare providers before having massage therapy to find out if any special precautions are needed. For instance, the application of deep or intense pressure is not recommended near cancer lesions or enlarged lymph nodes, radiation field sites, medical devices such as indwelling intravenous catheters (ports), or anatomic distortions such as postoperative changes, or in patients with a bleeding tendency. Since there are many types of massage to choose from—Swedish, shiatsu, reflexology, just to name a few—find out what type of massage may be best for you.

Evidence suggests that mindfulness-based stress reduction, a type of meditation training, can help cancer patients relieve anxiety, stress, fatigue, and general mood and sleep disturbances. Mind-body modalities include yoga, meditation, tai chi, hypnosis, relaxation techniques, and music therapy. You won't know if any of them can help unless you try!

Preliminary evidence indicates that yoga may help to improve anxiety, depression, distress, and stress in people with cancer. It also may help to lessen fatigue in breast cancer patients and survivors. Unfortunately, only a small number of yoga studies in cancer patients have been completed, and the quality of some studies has been questioned. Because yoga involves physical activity, it's important to talk with your healthcare providers in advance to find out whether any aspects of yoga might be unsafe for you. These days, many types and levels of yoga practice are available in cities and town across America, so it shouldn't be too difficult to find a place that suits your needs.

Various studies suggest possible benefits of hypnosis, relaxation therapies, and biofeedback to help patients manage cancer symptoms and treat side effects.

Therapies based on a philosophy of bioenergy fields (Reiki, therapeutic touch, healing touch, polarity therapy, and external qigong) are safe and may provide some benefit for reducing stress and enhancing a patient's quality of life. There is limited evidence as to their efficacy for symptom management, including reducing pain and fatigue.

Support groups, supportive/expressive therapy, cognitive-behavioral therapy, and cognitive-behavioral stress management are recommended as part of a multidisciplinary approach to reduce anxiety, mood disturbance, chronic pain, and to improve quality of life.

More About Supplements

A dietary supplement is a product intended for ingestion that contains a vitamin, mineral, amino acid, herb or other botanical, and enzymes/other ingredients intended to add further nutritional value to one's diet. Most claims that refer to the benefits of dietary supplements are anecdotal. In fact, by law, manufacturers are not allowed to claim that their product will cure, treat, or prevent a disease.

Any claim of benefits for some supplements may be supported by early research in a laboratory using cultured cells or lab animals. However, research studies looking for the same benefits in actual patients are very few and usually include only a few participants. This makes it difficult to generalize any benefits to a larger patient population.

Studies on whether herbal supplements—or substances derived from them—might be of value in cancer treatment are in their early stages, so scientific evidence is limited. Herbal supplements may have side effects, and some may interact in harmful ways with drugs, including drugs used in cancer treatment.

The effects of taking vitamin and mineral supplements, including antioxidant supplements, during cancer treatment are uncertain. NCI advises cancer patients to talk to their healthcare providers before taking any supplements.

A 2008 review of the research literature on herbal supplements and cancer concluded that although several herbs have shown promise for managing side effects and symptoms, such as nausea and vomiting, pain, fatigue, and insomnia, the scientific evidence is limited, and many clinical trials have not been well designed. Use of herbs for managing symptoms also raises concerns about potential negative interactions with conventional cancer treatments.

In addition, using supplements during chemotherapy or radiation therapy can be problematic because of drug–supplement interactions. For example, some herbs, such as ginkgo, garlic, ginger, bilberry, dong quai, feverfew, ginseng, turmeric, meadowsweet, and willow contain elements that possess antiplatelet activity. Others, such as chamomile, motherwort, horse chestnut, fenugreek, and red clover, contain coumarin, a chemical used in the synthesis of a number of synthetic blood thinners. Using these while taking anticoagulants (blood thinners) or prior to undergoing surgery can increase the risk of bleeding.

Liver toxicity may also be increased by using acetaminophen (Tylenol), along with the potentially liver-toxic herbs echinacea and kava. Opioid analgesics along with the sedative herbal supplements valerian, kava, and chamomile may lead to increased central nervous system (CNS) depression, and ginseng can sometimes inhibit the pain relief effect of opioids.

Patients on tamoxifen should not use red clover, dong quai, or licorice because they contain phytoestrogen (plant estrogen) components. St. John's wort, used by some for depression, can interfere with the metabolism of certain chemotherapy drugs, making them less effective.

These examples point out the importance of honest communications between you and your doctor about any dietary supplements you may be considering. If he or she is not adequately knowledgeable about the use of supplements, simply ask for a referral to someone in your area who can guide you appropriately.

Olivia Newton-John: East Meets West

Singer-actress Olivia Newton-John, diagnosed with cancer in 1992, also used complementary treatments, such as herbal supplements, acupuncture, meditation, and visualization. "I researched a lot and felt satisfied with my course of treatment. It was sort of an East meets West approach. I meditated every day, did yoga, used homeopathy, ate well—I boosted my inner strength as much as I could. When bad thoughts came in, I pushed them right out."[42]

Buyer Beware

Some products or practices advocated for cancer treatment may interfere with conventional cancer treatments or have other risks. You should consult your healthcare providers before using any complementary health approach. *None of them have cured cancer or caused it to go into remission.*

For example, a 2010 NCCIH-supported trial of a standardized shark cartilage extract, taken in addition to chemotherapy and radiation therapy, showed no benefit in patients with advanced lung cancer. An earlier, smaller study in patients with advanced breast or colorectal cancers also showed no benefit from the addition of shark cartilage to conventional treatment.

A 2011 systematic review of research on laetrile found no evidence that it is effective as a cancer treatment. Laetrile can be toxic, especially if taken orally, because it contains cyanide.

The FDA and the Federal Trade Commission (FTC) have warned the public to be aware of fraudulent cancer treatments. While these scams aren't new, in recent years it has become easier to market them to the public using the Internet.

---

42. *http://ww5.komen.org/BreastCancer/OliviaNewtonJohn.html#sthash.WLrKG1i8.dpuf*

Some fraudulent cancer treatments are harmful by themselves, and others can be indirectly harmful because people may delay seeking medical care while they try them, or because the fraudulent product interferes with the effectiveness of proven cancer treatments.

Scientific breakthrough!

Get your miraculous cure today!

Secret ingredients to cure you now!

Ancient remedy for today's diseases!

Treats all forms of cancer!

Shrinks malignant tumors instantly!

Recognize any of these advertising pitches? The people who sell fraudulent cancer treatments often market them with claims like these. The advertisements may include personal stories from people who've taken the product, but such stories—real or not—aren't reliable evidence that a product is effective. And a money-back guarantee does not provide proof that a product works.

If you're considering using any anticancer product you've seen in an advertisement, talk to your healthcare provider first. Additional information on cancer-related health frauds is available from the FDA[43] and the FTC.[44]

MY JOURNEY

I've always been interested in dietary supplements and have had good results with a steady regimen of vitamins and minerals, as well as the occasional extra for temporary ailments. So when I got cancer, I figured I would boost my intake and expand my menu to help

---

43. *http://www.fda.gov/ForConsumers/ConsumerUpdates/ucm048383.htm*
44. *http://www.ftc.gov/bcp/edu/pubs/consumer/alerts/alt079.pdf*

fight the disease, especially during chemotherapy treatments. I did my research and started with glutamine to aid digestion and relieve mouth sores, maitake mushrooms to shrink the tumor, and fish oil to reduce inflammation. But when I shared this with my oncologist, he held up his hand right away, as if to say STOP! He explained his concern about studies showing that these may interfere with the chemo drugs doing their work. While I respect my doctor, I'm not sure he knows enough about these options. At the same time, can I believe everything I read online? Since both answers are probably a resounding *no*, I am still figuring out what to do or who else I can talk to.

Malik (Baltimore, Maryland)

Low-Dose Chemotherapy

While traditional chemotherapy is normally prescribed in potent doses, metronomic chemotherapy involves the use of lower doses of chemotherapy administered more frequently and regularly, such as weekly or daily. This is in contrast with conventional treatments, which are given at maximum tolerated levels every three weeks at doses just below what have proven to cause over 50 percent of patients to experience severe or dose-limiting toxicity.

Low-dose chemo is intended to ease the burden on a patient, especially when used with naturopathic remedies, which include nutritional and physiological therapies. When combined, these synergistic approaches have been associated with improved treatment consistency, duration, and outcome. These anticancer effects are due to the following elements:

- Anti-angiogenesis
- Improving anticancer immune responses by suppressing immune regulatory cells

- Killing more chemo-sensitive cycling cancer cells
- Less tumor cell recovery time between treatments
- Less likelihood of encountering tumor chemoresistance

Dr. Judah Folkman, former professor at Harvard University and director of the vascular biology program at Children's Hospital Boston, was the first major proponent of the potential for metronomic chemotherapy in the 1990s, and he inspired many oncologists to explore these methods.

For example, Nick Chen is a leading medical oncologist and founder of the Seattle Integrative Cancer Center. According to Ralph W. Moss, PhD, a founding advisor to the National Institute of Health's Office of Alternative Medicine (now the NCCAM) and advisor to Breast Cancer Action and the Susan G. Komen Breast Cancer Foundation, "Nick Chen is the rare medical oncologist who recognizes the importance of nutritional, mental and emotional health in cancer." When it comes to integrative oncology, Moss says that, "I have seen the future, and it works. As a resident of a part of the country where naturopathy is not even licensed, I cast envious eyes on the Pacific Northwest, whose residents have far greater options when it comes to the varieties of treatment they can access. I think those who fear the sky will fall if they license naturopathy should study how well it works in states such as Oregon and Washington, where naturopathy has been accepted since the 1920s."

Dr. Chen presents a persuasive case for giving drugs metronomically (in low doses) in conjunction with naturopathic post-care, which he has seen yield remarkable results in certain cancers. Patient results have also been positive.

Bickley Barich was diagnosed with stage IV metastatic ovarian cancer, and after three years of treatment with heavy chemotherapy, her oncologist told her there was nothing more he could do. Metronomic chemotherapy proved to be more effective than her previous treatments, and this integrative approach has given her ten years (and counting) with her family.

After twelve years with very advanced prostate cancer, Dr. Samuel Mahaffy is now thriving, due in large part a treatment program of metronomic chemotherapy in combination with naturopathic medicine.

We suggest that you investigate these possibilities with your oncologist and see if they are a viable option for you and the particular type of cancer you are treating.

Marijuana and Cancer

Cannabis, also known as marijuana, is a plant that originated in Central Asia and is grown in many parts of the world today, including here in America, although it is still illegal to do so in most states.

The cannabis plant produces a resin containing compounds called cannabinoids. Some are psychoactive, which act on the brain and change mood or consciousness. In the United States, cannabis is a controlled substance and has been classified as a Schedule I agent (a drug with increased potential for abuse and no known medical use).

Cannabinoids are active chemicals in cannabis that cause drug-like effects throughout the body, including the central nervous system and the immune system. The main active cannabinoid in cannabis is delta-9-THC. Another active cannabinoid is cannabidiol (CBD), which may relieve pain and lower inflammation without causing the "high" of delta-9-THC.

What many people do not know is that our bodies make cannabinoids called endocannabinoids. Many of these are present in the human body; however, the two most common are AEA and 2-AG. Although they may not have the same psychoactive effects as the

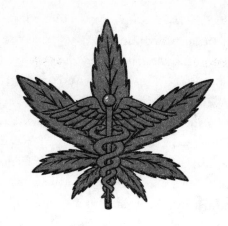

Medical Marijuana
Source: Larry Rains (*istock.com*)

cannabinoids in marijuana, they still play a key role as a modulator in the functions of neurologic and immune system pathways.

Endocannabinoids exert their effects by binding to specific receptors on their target cells. There are two main types of cannabinoid receptors, CB1 and CB2. CB1 receptors are found mostly in nerve cells (neurons) in the central and peripheral nervous system, while CB2 receptors are most commonly identified in the immune cells.

In addition to cannabinoids, marijuana smoke contains many of the same chemical components as tobacco smoke, including arsenic, benzene, formaldehyde, and lead, all of which are known carcinogens. Although it does not contain nicotine, marijuana smoke does contain ammonia, carbon monoxide, hydrogen cyanide, and tar.

Possible effects of cannabinoids include anti-inflammatory activity, antiviral activity, as well as the ability to block cell growth, prevent the growth of blood vessels that supply tumors, and relieve muscle spasms caused by multiple sclerosis.

Cannabis may be taken by mouth or inhaled. When taken orally (in baked products or as an herbal tea), the main psychoactive ingredient (delta-9-THC) is processed by the liver, which makes an additional psychoactive chemical. Unfortunately, studies of the absorption of THC through the stomach can be slow and erratic, leading to varying amounts in the blood. THC can also be broken down by acid in the stomach.

When cannabis smoke is inhaled, cannabinoids quickly enter the bloodstream. THC is detectable in the blood within seconds and peaks within ten minutes. Another method of inhalation is called vaporization, which uses a device commonly targeted for e-cigarettes. In vaporization, marijuana is heated to a temperature between 180° and 200° C. This releases the active ingredients but only trace amounts of a few other chemicals. It is said to remove approximately 95 percent of the smoke that would otherwise be inhaled.

By federal law, the use, sale, and possession of cannabis (marijuana) are forbidden in the United States. However, a growing number of states (twenty-three) and the District of Columbia have enacted laws to legalize *medical* marijuana.

Musician Melissa Etheridge used medicinal marijuana during her chemotherapy treatments for breast cancer and says she's continued using it ever since to help cope with the lingering side effects she experiences from the high doses of chemotherapy. In a guest column for CNN, she shared her thoughts on how marijuana helped her. "People use marijuana for different reasons, and I needed it to get me through tough times. I used it every day during chemo: It gave me an appetite so I was able to eat and keep my strength up. It also helped with the depression, and it eased gastrointestinal pain, even to this day. I even find it helps with regulating my sleep."

Pharmaceutical Cannabinoids and the FDA

Two synthetic forms of cannabinoid are approved by the FDA and can be legally prescribed. Dronabinol, available in capsule form, is approved by the FDA to treat chemotherapy-induced nausea and vomiting (CINV) and anorexia associated with weight loss in patients with AIDS.

The second form, nabilone, is approved by the FDA only for CINV. It is also a capsule. The main limitation to both of these drugs is that taking a capsule may be difficult for patients with nausea/vomiting.

One other cannabinol of note is called nabiximol. It is a whole-plant extract of marijuana and contains a ratio of THC to CBD as 1.08:1.00. It is used as an oral mucosal spray and is currently approved for use in Canada and parts of Europe. It is in clinical trials in the United States.

MY JOURNEY

I have been serving as a minister of God for most of my life. I have been taught to believe that God is our healer and that medicine must be used only in times of complete and total emergency.

Recently, one of my congregants began treatment for cancer, and she was experiencing terrible headaches as a result of the chemotherapy she was receiving. As much as I did not agree with her choice, on religious grounds, it was hard to argue with the scientific fact that the tumor was shrinking. But the headaches were becoming debilitating, and one of her doctors advised her to try medical marijuana. She came to me asking for my advice. I was torn, as this is not normally something I would even consider, but upon further reflection and prayer, I came to realize that this is a plant, which grows naturally from God's earth, and if it will relieve this woman's headaches and allow her to be a more effective wife and mother, who am I to stop her?

Anonymous (Seattle, Washington)

Treating Cancer with Cannabinoids

Cannabinoid receptors have been found on cancer cells, and they have been shown to have some antitumor effects.[45] Studies in mice and rats have shown that cannabinoids may inhibit tumor growth by causing cell death, blocking cell growth, and blocking the development of blood vessels needed by tumors to grow. Other animal studies have shown that cannabinoids may kill cancer cells while protecting normal cells.

Clinical trials in patients, however, have been extremely limited. For this reason, there are no current recommendations for the use of marijuana in the direct treatment of cancer.

Tommy Chong: Using Marijuana to Treat His Cancers

Canadian comedian, actor, writer, director, activist, and former *Dancing with the Stars* contestant, Tommy Chong told *US Weekly* in June 2015 that he had been diagnosed with rectal cancer. In true Cheech and Chong fashion, he tweeted, "I have good news and bad news. First the bad news, the cancer came back and it's a real pain in the butt."

In an interview with *Access Hollywood Live*, Chong said that he sought medical advice when he began to experience blood in his stool and was told that his cancer was in stage I. He said he would undergo a short course of chemotherapy and radiation therapy before having the tumor removed surgically, which he did in October 2015.

This is not Chong's first time dealing with cancer. Three years earlier, he was diagnosed with cancer of the prostate. As a vocal marijuana-legalization advocate, Chong used cannabis oil (as a suppository) to treat his cancer and smoked marijuana to relieve some of his symptoms.

---

45. Joan L. Kramer, MD, CA, "Medical Marijuana for Cancer," *A Cancer Journal for Clinicians*, Vol. 65, no. 2, Mar/Apr 2015: 109–122.

"I'm using cannabis like crazy now," he told *US Weekly* at the time. "More so than ever before. I'm in treatment now, and either I get healed or I don't. But either way, I'm going to make sure I get a little edge off or put up."

Using Medical Marijuana to Treat Side Effects

While its potential to treat cancer as a disease is yet to be determined, medical marijuana has already proven to be beneficial for many cancer patients in treating some of the side effects of treatment:

- Chemotherapy-induced nausea and vomiting (CINV)
- Poor appetite and weight loss
- Pain
- Anxiety
- Sleep deprivation

Despite advances in pharmacologic and nonpharmacological management, nausea and vomiting (N/V) remain distressing side effects for cancer patients and their families. As previously mentioned, both dronabinol and nabilone are now approved by the FDA for the treatment of chemotherapy-induced nausea and vomiting.

Let's look at how medical marijuana might treat the above side effects of cancer treatments, as well as some side effects of cannabinoids.

Chemotherapy-Induced Nausea and Vomiting (CINV)

Several studies are looking at smoked marijuana and CINV. In one review of over 1,300 patients, cannabinoids were found to be more effective than conventional antiemetics, such as prochlorperazine, metoclopramide, chlorpromazine, thiethylperazine, haloperidol, domperidone, and alizapride. However, reported side effects included a feeling of being high, euphoria, drowsiness, dizziness, depression, hallucinations, paranoia, and hypotension (low blood pressure).

Poor Appetite and Weight Loss

Anorexia, early satiety, weight loss, and cachexia are common problems for cancer patients. Some are faced not only with the disfigurement associated with these symptoms but also with the inability to engage in the social interaction of meals.

Perhaps not surprisingly, trials conducted in the 1980s that involved healthy control subjects showed that inhaling marijuana led to an increase in caloric intake, mainly in the form of between-meal snacks, with increased intakes of fatty and sweet foods. The question is, would this effect also be seen in cancer patients?

Three controlled trials demonstrated that oral THC has variable effects on appetite stimulation and weight loss in patients with advanced malignancies and human immunodeficiency virus (HIV) infection. Some studies showed increased appetite, but weight gain did not necessarily accompany the improvement in appetite. One study showed that dronabinol could improve altered taste sensations associated with chemotherapy.

Pain

Cancer pain results from inflammation, invasion of bone or other pain-sensitive structures, or nerve injury. When cancer pain is severe and persistent, it is often resistant to treatment with opioids. Managing or, in some cases, even relieving pain, which medical marijuana has been shown to do, improves a patient's quality of life through all stages of cancer.

Two studies examined the effects of oral delta-9-THC on cancer pain. The first, a double-blind, placebo-controlled study involving ten patients, measured both pain intensity and pain relief.[46] It was reported that 15 mg and 20 mg doses of the cannabinoid delta-9-THC were

---

46. http://www.ncbi.nlm.nih.gov/pubmed/1091664?dopt=Abstract

associated with substantial analgesic effects, with antiemetic effects, and appetite stimulation.

Another study[47] examined the effects of a plant extract with controlled cannabinoid content in an oromucosal spray. In a multicenter, double-blind, placebo-controlled study, the THC:CBD nabiximols extract and THC extract alone were compared in the analgesic management of patients with advanced cancer and with moderate-to-severe cancer-related pain. The researchers concluded that the THC:CBD extract was efficacious for pain relief in advanced cancer patients whose pain was not fully relieved by strong opioids.

Anxiety

A small number of studies have shown that the use of cannabinoid delta-9-THC is associated with a reduction in a patient's anxiety. Depending on their previous familiarity, patients often experience mood elevation after exposure to cannabis. In a five-patient case series of inhaled cannabis that examined analgesic effects in chronic pain, it was reported that patients who self-administered cannabis had improved mood and sense of well-being and less anxiety.

Sleep Deprivation

One small placebo-controlled study of dronabinol in cancer patients noted an increased quality of sleep and relaxation in those treated with THC. Another common effect of cannabis is sleepiness. A small placebo-controlled study of dronabinol in cancer patients with altered chemosensory perception also noted an increased quality of sleep and relaxation in those treated with THC.

---

47. *http://www.ncbi.nlm.nih.gov/pubmed/19896326?dopt=Abstract*

The Flip Side: Adverse Effects

Because cannabinoid receptors, unlike opioid receptors, are not located in the brainstem areas controlling respiration, lethal overdoses from cannabis and cannabinoids do *not* occur. However, cannabinoid receptors are present in other tissues throughout the body, not just in the central nervous system, and adverse effects include rapid heartbeat, low blood pressure, red eyes, muscle relaxation, and slowed gastrointestinal motility.

Although cannabinoids are considered by some to be addictive drugs, their addictive potential is considerably lower than that of other prescribed agents or substances of abuse. The brain, however, can develop a tolerance to cannabinoids.

Withdrawal symptoms such as irritability, insomnia with sleep electroencephalogram disturbance, restlessness, hot flashes, and, rarely, nausea and cramping have been observed. However, these symptoms appear to be mild compared with withdrawal symptoms associated with opiates or benzodiazepines, and the symptoms usually dissipate after a few days.

Since cannabis smoke contains many of the same components as tobacco smoke, there are valid concerns about the adverse pulmonary effects of inhaled cannabis. Marijuana smoke can cause injury to the lungs and airways, but there is no clear link to marijuana smoke and the development of chronic obstructive pulmonary disease (COPD). Many of the effects of marijuana smoke subside after marijuana use has stopped.

NOTE to PATIENT:
For more information, visit *www.reimaginingcancer.com*.

Bringing Mind and Body Together

Cancer centers throughout the country are discovering that providing genuine, lasting wellness for their patients may require more than the traditional methods they have offered in the past. As a result, they are incorporating a menu of new options that complement and expand existing methods of treatment. These new offerings generally focus on the multiple benefits of connecting the mind and body—as a tool to combat side effects, as a method for better communication between patients and doctors, and as a viable means for patients to express and process the many levels of vulnerability that any diagnosis of cancer creates.

For example, patient services in many cancer centers now offer art therapy that may include painting and sculpture classes, dance, theater, and writing programs. Each of these has proven to be a remarkable opportunity for patients (and caregivers) to relieve stress while providing outlets for much-needed personal expression.

Writing, in particular, seems to offer multiple possibilities for patients to explore their feelings as well as to document their experience for pragmatic purposes. According to Nancy Morgan, a writing clinician and director of the Georgetown Lombardi Comprehensive Cancer Center Arts & Humanities program in Washington, DC, "Twenty years of research in controlled laboratory settings indicates writing may contribute to improved physical and emotional health . . . we found that just one writing session in a busy cancer clinic where the patients are frequently interrupted can still have a positive impact on patients."[48]

Morgan's studies suggest a strong possibility that writing down one's thoughts and feelings can change a patient's view of their cancer, opening up another door to improving their quality of life, even from a physical perspective.

---

48. *The Oncologist*, February 2008

Many patients reported that, although they don't necessarily like talking about cancer, writing about it certainly helped them get through it.[49]

Bruce D. Cheson, MD, a coauthor on the study, reported that, "Many of our patients were interested in this kind of therapy. Our study supports the benefit of an expressive writing program and the ability to integrate such a program into a busy clinic."

―――――――――――― MY JOURNEY ――――――――――――

I've never been a good student or anything like that, and never kept a journal or even wrote many emails, and I don't text very much except to my children because that's the only way they actually communicate. But when I got cancer and started treatment, I had so many thoughts running through my head all the time that I had to do something to calm myself down and get focused. Writing really helped my mind stop racing so much, and I even get less scared and stuff from writing about how I feel. And, of course, writing down things I need to do is very practical because cancer means having a lot of extra stuff to remember, with all the damn appointments and medicines and everything else. I used to go to my doctor and forget most of what I wanted to ask her, but when I write down my questions, it makes a huge difference. Now if I can only remember to bring the paper with me, I'll be all set.

Bob (Brooklyn, New York)

Put It in Writing

What if you began expressing yourself in writing, and that led you to communicate more effectively with your family, friends, and

―――――――――――――――――――――――――――――――――――

49. *Coping with Cancer*, March/April 2009

doctors? What if writing relieved some of your stress and helped you feel more in control of your situation? What if other people in your life became inspired by how you began coping with your challenges?

"Who am I?" touches us on spiritual and pragmatic levels. It can be both an existential and a moment-by-moment question. In times of great change and stress, such as in response to a diagnosis of cancer, we will question our sense of self, and the ways in which we previously identified ourselves may be turned upside down. Whether you are a patient or a caregiver of any kind, it's vital that you see life with clear eyes, and that begins each morning when you look in the mirror. If you've been diagnosed with cancer, you're probably facing enormous challenges and need to focus a great deal on yourself. If you are a patient's caretaker, doctor, or nurse—responsible for someone else's health—you also need to take care of yourself. Writing can help. You can begin with two simple exercises and *no* rules. You're the boss of you, not your high school English teacher.

The first is called, "I AM" and asks you to listen to the core of your mind and body. Start with those two words—I AM—and just write whatever comes to mind. It may be emotional or philosophical or physical or all three somehow combined. There are no wrong answers! But there are compelling reasons for getting in touch with yourself, especially when your very existence is being challenged.

The second exercise involves writing a simple "To Do" list. If you or someone you care about has been diagnosed with cancer, that list has suddenly expanded with an entirely new set of protocols to handle, from keeping track of doctors' appointments and medication regimens to communicating with family, friends, and colleagues about how cancer—directly or indirectly—is affecting your life. That can be daunting, so do yourself a favor and get organized. Write down what you need to do and when, whom you want to talk to and how you wish to approach them. Each To Do item on the list is bound to beg for more. But more is good. It means you're getting things done, including the challenging tasks you may ordinarily avoid.

Let your list encourage you to live in the moment and guide you bravely into an uncertain future. Take a few minutes to write down the small things, and, while you're at it, take a stab at the big issues, too. Surprises are waiting with each step you take.[50]

And While You're At It—The Healing Power of Laughter

If you could bottle laughter and offer it for sale, pharmacies all over the world would be selling it like hotcakes and turning into palaces. I mean, what feels better than laughing?

We've all heard the saying, "Laughter is the best medicine." We've also heard endless claims from self-proclaimed healers, traveling salesmen, and websites about holistic, organic cures for everything under the sun. As far as we know, only three things exist that contain the therapeutic qualities needed to cure anything: love, positivity, and laughter. Without these three, even the strongest medicine may not do the trick.

When things are bad; when the fear is great and the treatments are harsh; when you're puking all night and your hair falls out; when your wife goes bald or your husband goes limp; when your patience fails or you just don't know what to do, how in God's name are you to survive—even for another day?

Laughter. We were born with this gift. It can elevate our spirits and make us happy. Laughter is contagious, too. It brings people together. If you get on a good roll, you'll feel stronger and more alive, no matter what shape you're in or how bad you feel.

Norman Cousins, a former editor at the *Saturday Review*, put the concept of laugh therapy on the map in 1976 when his article in the

---

50. From David Tabatsky, *Write for Life: Communicating Your Way Through Cancer* (2013).

New England Journal of Medicine described how he had been afflicted with a rare degenerative disease of the connective tissue. After suffering a series of setbacks in the hospital, he decided to check into a hotel, take massive doses of vitamin C, watch Marx Brothers movies, and read funny books for days on end. Eventually, his symptoms abated and most of the freedom of movement he had lost he regained. Cousins beautifully told his story of the power of the mind on the body in his book *Anatomy of an Illness* (Norton, 1979). Although no one in the medical community can say for sure what essentially cured Cousins, his story does seem to suggest that love, positivity, and laughter can be effective allies in the fight against disease.

How do you have fun? What makes you laugh? Can you describe three things that make you laugh? Of course, no one will stop you if you don't end at three and keep going, and that is definitely encouraged.

For people living with cancer, it may seem strange or even distasteful to consider humor when facing such serious issues. Yet laughter can be helpful in ways you might not have realized or imagined. Laughter can help you feel better about yourself and the world around you. Have you looked at the world lately? It's pretty funny. Then again, it's pretty sad, and we need comic relief—lots of it.

Laughter is a natural diversion. When you laugh, no other thought comes to mind. Laughing can also induce physical changes in the body. After laughing for just a few minutes, you may feel better for hours. When used to supplement conventional cancer treatments, laughter therapy may help in the overall healing process. According to some studies, laughter therapy may provide physical benefits, such as boosting the immune system and circulatory system; enhancing oxygen intake; stimulating the heart and lungs; relaxing muscles throughout the body; triggering the release of endorphins (the body's natural painkillers); easing digestion, soothing stomachaches, and relieving pain; balancing blood pressure; and improving mental functions (alertness, memory, creativity).

Laughter therapy may also improve overall attitude, reduce stress and tension, promote relaxation, aid sleep, enhance quality of life, strengthen social bonds and relationships, and produce a general sense of well-being.

In fact, some cancer centers have started support groups dedicated to creating laughter as part of their mind-body wellness programs. It's a form of physical and emotional therapy that helps patients cope while receiving conventional cancer treatments. According to many participants, they were able to leave their troubles at the door and stop thinking about cancer. Instead, they learned that even while dealing with what sometimes may feel like an insurmountable challenge, they *can* still laugh and even feel better.

Sounds like just what the doctor ordered.[51]

Mandy Patinkin: "Be Happy"

Maybe you know him from his portrayal of Che in Andrew Lloyd Webber's *Evita*, or as Jason Gideon on *Criminal Minds*, or Saul Berenson in the Showtime series *Homeland*. Most people, however, recognize actor Mandy Patinkin as the sword-wielding Inigo Montoya in the 1987 movie *The Princess Bride*, with his mantra: *"Hello, my name is Inigo Montoya. You killed my father. Prepare to die."*

In 2004, at the age of fifty-one, the same age at which his father died from pancreatic cancer, Patinkin was diagnosed with prostate cancer and successfully treated with radical prostatectomy.

As he told *Coping with Cancer*, he is a survivor who is conscientious about maintaining his health. He drinks antioxidant-rich smoothies and eats at least one of these five foods—broccoli, cauliflower,

---

51. From Tabatsky, *Write for Life*.

Brussels sprouts, blueberries, and cooked tomatoes—every day, as they are thought to help fight cancer. He keeps his stress levels low with a regimen of daily meditation, exercise, quality time with his family, and philanthropy. His current mantra is simply "Be happy."

"And I'm so very aware," he said, "as I never was before cancer, that I may live to 100. I hope I do. I probably will never die from prostate cancer; I don't have a prostate anymore. But I know that life could be over in five seconds, or fifty minutes, or fifty years. I just hope I get fifty years rather than fifty minutes."[52]

---

52. *http://copingmag.com/cwc/index.php/celebrities/celebrity_article/mandy_patinkin*

KEY POINTS TO REMEMBER

✓ Save your energy and balance rest with activity.

✓ Eat and drink well, and seek nutritional counseling.

✓ Tell your doctor about *all* medicines you are taking, including herbs, vitamins, and supplements.

✓ Palliative care is not specifically end-of-life care. It offers you a plan to manage pain and can be quite temporary.

✓ Keep track of your pain profile. Take pain medicine as prescribed by your doctor.

✓ Tell your doctor about problems that interfere with sleep, and set good bedtime habits.

✓ Cancer patients receiving integrative therapies in the hospital may have less pain and anxiety.

✓ Massage therapy may lead to short-term improvements in pain and mood in patients with cancer.

✓ Yoga and other mind-body practices may help lessen anxiety, depression, and stress.

✓ Acupuncture can help cancer patients manage treatment-related nausea and vomiting.

✓ Read the fine print! If you're considering using any anticancer product you've seen advertised, talk to your healthcare provider first.

✓ Medical marijuana has proven to be beneficial for many cancer patients in treating some of the side effects of treatment.

WHAT CANCER CANNOT DO

Cancer is so limited . . .
It cannot cripple love.
It cannot shatter hope.
It cannot corrode faith.
It cannot eat away peace.
It cannot destroy confidence.
It cannot kill friendship.
It cannot shut out memories.
It cannot silence courage.

It cannot reduce eternal life.

10 SAVE YOUR OWN LIFE: How to Prevent Cancer or Catch It Early

Cancer is one big bully.
But if we all stand up to cancer together,
we can kick its ass so good, it'll never come back.

—Samuel L. Jackson

Bad Luck or Bad Environment?

In January 2015, renowned cancer researcher Bert Vogelstein of Johns Hopkins University School of Medicine published a study suggesting that developing certain types of cancer is just the result of "bad luck." Some people in the field interpreted his work to mean that screening and early detection might be more important than preventing cancer from developing in the first place. This spin on Dr. Vogelstein's data was so controversial that it created a firestorm of clashing views about how much time, effort, and money we should spend trying to prevent the disease if, indeed, developing cancer is mostly the result of bad luck.

One year later, in January 2016, a group of researchers from Stony Brook University published a study that came to the opposite conclusion, declaring that most cancers are caused by factors in our environments and can therefore be prevented. Here's the Stony Brook list of preventable cancers and the factors that cause them.

Cancer Type	Preventable Risk	Risk Factors
Anus	>63%	HPV infection, smoking
Colon & rectum	>75%	Diet, smoking, alcohol, obesity
Esophagus	>75%	Smoking, alcohol, obesity, diet
Head & Neck	>75%	Tobacco & alcohol
Kidney	>58%	Smoking, obesity, workplace exposures
Liver	~80%	Hepatitis B and C virus infections
Lung	>90%	Smoking, air pollution
Lymphoma	>71%	Chemicals, radiation, immune system deficiency
Mouth & voice box	~70%	HPV infection
Prostate	Substantial	Diet, smoking, obesity
Skin—melanoma	65–86%	Sun exposure
Skin—basal cell	~90%	Ultraviolet (UV) radiation
Stomach	65–80%	*Helicobacter pylori* infection
Thyroid	>72%	Diet low in iodine, radiation

> means "greater than"
~ means "approximately equal to"

So who's right, Dr. Vogelstein or the Stony Brook scientists?
They both are.

At its root, cancer is a disease of your DNA. You inherit your DNA from your parents, and it really is a matter of luck which combinations of genes you end up with. If some of these genes can cause cancer or just make you more likely to develop certain types (as described in Chapter 3), knowing your family medical history, screening, and early detection will be the main tools for saving your life.

However, most cancers are not caused by inherited genes but by damage to your DNA that occurs in your lifetime. As the Stony Brook researchers pointed out, depending on the type of cancer, we can reduce our risk of developing cancer by 60 to 90 percent through changes in our lifestyles and environment.

Environment and Lifestyle Factors

For many years, researchers have been studying several different ways to help prevent cancer. Considering some factors, the evidence is conclusive, while for others things are not so clear. The following table shows some of the risk factors/exposures that possess ample evidence linking them to cancer.

Risk Factor	Examples	Preventable Cancers
Cigarette smoking and Tobacco	Cigarettes, smokeless tobacco	Acute myelogenous leukemia (AML) Bladder Esophagus Kidney Lung Mouth and tongue Pancreas Stomach

Infections	HPV	Cervix, penis, vagina, anus, oral
	Hepatitis B and C	Liver
	Epstein-Barr Virus	Burkitt's lymphoma
	Helicobacter pylori	Stomach
	HIV-AIDS	Kaposi sarcoma
Radiation	UV radiation	Skin cancers
	Ionizing radiation	Leukemia, thyroid, breast
Drugs that suppress the immune system	Transplant patients	Non-Hodgkin lymphoma (NHL), lung, kidney, liver

A number of factors may affect the risk of cancer, but the overall evidence among them is not as strong. These factors include diet, alcohol, physical activity, obesity, and diabetes. It is hard to study the effects of diet on cancer because your diet may include both foods that protect against cancer as well as foods that may increase the risk of cancer. It is also hard for participants in studies to keep track of what they eat over a long period of time. This may be one explanation why studies looking at the effect of diet on cancer risk can have different results.

Other lifestyle factors are also hard to study. It is common knowledge that people who are physically active have a lower risk of certain cancers than those who are not, but it is not known if physical activity itself is the reason for this. And although it is known that those with obesity have a higher rate of cancer, we don't know whether losing weight decreases that risk.

The role of diabetes in cancer is further complicated by the fact that many of the risk factors that cause diabetes (diet, obesity, lack of activity, and smoking) also affect one's cancer risk. It is hard to know whether the risk of cancer is increased more by diabetes or by these risk factors themselves. Studies are underway to see how medicine that is used to treat diabetes affects cancer risk.

This table outlines these factors that *may* affect the risk of cancer. Arrows pointing up indicate a possible increased risk, while arrows pointing down indicate the possibility of a decreased risk.

Risk Factor	↑/↓	Cancer
Diet		
Fruit and non-starchy vegetables	↓	Oral cancer
		Esophageal cancer
		Stomach cancer
Fruit	↓	Lung cancer
Diet high in fat, protein, red meat	↑/↓	Colorectal cancer
Low fat, high fiber, high fruits and vegetables.	↓	Colorectal cancer
Alcohol	↑	Oral cancer
	↑	Esophageal cancer
	↑	Breast cancer
	↑	Colorectal cancer (in men)
	↑	Liver and colorectal cancer (in women)
Physical activity	↓	Colorectal cancer
	↓	Postmenopausal breast cancer
	↓	Endometrial cancer
Obesity	↑	Postmenopausal breast cancer
	↑	Colorectal cancer
	↑	Endometrial cancer
	↑	Esophageal cancer
	↑	Kidney cancer

Obesity *(continued)*	↑	Pancreatic cancer
	↑	Cancer of the gallbladder
Diabetes	↑	Bladder cancer
	↑	Breast cancer in women
	↑	Colorectal cancer
	↑	Endometrial cancer
	↑	Liver cancer
	↑	Lung cancer
	↑	Oral cancer
	↑	Oropharyngeal cancer
	↑	Ovarian cancer
	↑	Pancreatic cancer
Environmental Risk Factors		
Air pollution, second hand smoke, asbestos	↑	Lung cancer
Arsenic in drinking water	↑	Skin cancer
	↑	Bladder cancer
	↑	Lung cancer

But I Did Everything Right!

For anyone with cancer, regardless of gender, the shock of the diagnosis is often accompanied with bewilderment that this could have happened to someone who faithfully followed the rules of healthy living.

Gill Deacon, one of Canada's best-known environmental writers and a virtual poster child for mindful living and sustainable consumption, is one of those people. She was diagnosed with cancer at the age of forty-two, and it came as a slap in the face to someone who, according to her, "measured carbon emissions, rode her bike in the rain, said no to high fructose corn syrup and yes to rabbit food."

In her memoir *Naked Imperfection* (Penguin Canada, 2014), Gill writes about her cancer experience and how she came to realize that her "lifestyle wasn't an antidote to misfortune."

Gill's story is one of an overachiever who had lived her whole life trying to maintain control and attain various ideals of perfection. She approached cancer as "the newest challenge to be met, survival just one more thing to achieve." Gill eventually came to the realization that cancer is not just something else she can control and that the outcome is not entirely in her hands. Fortunately, her outcome has been positive and she now regards cancer as a gift—albeit one wrapped in barbed wire—that has given her new perspective on life.

Chemoprevention Strategies for Prostate Cancer

Chemoprevention refers to the use of substances to lower the risk of cancer or keep it from recurring. The substances may be natural or made in a laboratory. Some chemopreventive agents are tested in people who are at high risk for a certain type of cancer. The risk may be because of a precancerous condition, family history, or lifestyle factors.

Several factors make prostate cancer a prime candidate in the search for chemopreventive agents: the high incidence of the disease; the potentially long latency period between early dysplastic changes and invasive cancer; the tumor's dependency on androgens; and the ability to distinguish intermediate stages, or endpoints, for use in clinical trials. Even if a chemopreventive agent is unable to reverse premalignant disease, delaying the progression to invasive cancer may be sufficient to significantly improve survival and avoid complications from treatment.

As discussed in Chapter 2, androgens are a type of hormone that promotes the development and maintenance of male sex characteristics. Testosterone and dihydrotestosterone (DHT) are the most abundant androgens in men. Almost all testosterone is produced in the testicles, while a small amount is produced by the adrenal glands. Androgens promote the growth of prostate cells by binding to and activating the androgen receptor, a protein that is expressed in prostate cells. Once activated, the androgen receptor stimulates the expression of specific genes that cause prostate cells to grow.

Testosterone is converted into DHT (the most active androgen in the prostate) by the enzyme 5-alpha reductase (5-AR). Therefore, it makes sense that a drug that is able to inhibit this conversion may be useful in decreasing the growth of cells—both normal and cancerous —in the prostate.

Two 5-AR inhibitors have been closely looked at for this purpose. The drugs finasteride and dutasteride have been used for several years in the treatment of benign prostatic hypertrophy. They have also been studied as chemopreventive agents in clinical trials.

Finasteride blocks 5-AR, significantly decreasing DHT while leaving testosterone levels normal or slightly increased. A large trial, the Prostate Cancer Prevention Trial (PCPT),[53] tested finasteride as a chemopreventive agent. Almost 19,000 men considered to be at high risk were randomly selected to be treated with either finasteride or a placebo, and were followed for fifteen years. The results showed that although the finasteride-treated group showed a 25 percent lower incidence of prostate cancer, the overall survival rate of the two groups fifteen years later was nearly identical.

The ten-year survival rates for men diagnosed with prostate cancer during the trial period also showed no significant difference. The only

---

53. *http://www.cancer.gov/types/prostate/research/prostate-cancer-prevention-trial-qa*

somewhat troublesome finding from the trial was that when prostate cancer was diagnosed, the men who had received finasteride showed an increase in high-grade disease. High-grade tumors (Gleason score 7–10) are more likely to grow quickly and spread beyond the prostate than lower-grade tumors.

Dutasteride inhibits two types of 5-AR. It suppresses DHT by more than 90 percent but increases testosterone more than finasteride. A double-blind trial called REDUCE studied dutasteride. In the trial, 8,300 men considered to be at an increased risk of prostate cancer were randomly assigned to receive either dutasteride or a placebo for four years. The key findings showed that dutasteride significantly decreased the incidence of prostate cancer. But once again, there was no difference in prostate cancer or overall mortality. The reduction in prostate cancer incidence occurred primarily in less aggressive cancers (Gleason 5–6) and not in more aggressive cancers (Gleason 7–10), raising the question of whether this reduction in incidence would lead to any reduction in mortality.

What's the bottom line on these two drugs?

Guidelines from an expert panel of the American Society of Clinical Oncology (ASCO) and the American Urological Association (AUA)[54] advise that men who are considering a 5-AR inhibitor (5-ARI) for chemoprevention should know the following:

- Although the agents reduce the incidence of prostate cancer, they do not reduce the risk to zero.
- There may be an elevated risk of high-grade cancer with the use of a 5-ARI. The significance of this finding is presently unclear.
- No information on long-term effects of 5-ARIs is available.
- Whether 5-ARIs reduce prostate cancer mortality or increase life expectancy is currently unknown.

---

54. *https://www.auanet.org/education/guidelines/prostate-cancer-chemoprevention.cfm*

- Possible but reversible sexual side effects exist, including erectile dysfunction, loss of libido, and gynecomastia.
- 5-ARIs may improve lower urinary tract systems due to BPH.
- The FDA has reviewed the data of these studies and does not recommend them for use for chemoprevention.

The SELECT Trial

SELECT stands for the Selenium and Vitamin E Cancer Prevention Trial, a clinical trial to determine if one or both of these substances could help prevent prostate cancer when taken as dietary supplements. NCI primarily funded the trial. SWOG, an international network of research institutions, developed and conducted the trial. Over 35,000 men, age fifty and older at the start of the trial, participated and were randomly assigned to receive a daily dose of vitamin E and a placebo, selenium and a placebo, vitamin E and selenium, or two placebos.

The initial results of SELECT, published in 2009, showed no statistically significant differences in rates of prostate cancer in the four groups. The vitamin E–alone group demonstrated a nonsignificant increase in prostate cancer rates. The selenium-alone group showed a nonsignificant increase in diabetes mellitus. Based on those findings, the data and safety monitoring committee recommended that the trial be stopped early and that participants stop taking the study supplements.

In 2011, when researchers updated the information, they discovered that, compared with a placebo, the rate of prostate cancer detection was now significantly greater in the vitamin E–alone group and represented a 17 percent increase in prostate cancer risk. The study revealed a greater incidence of prostate cancer in men who had taken selenium than in men who had taken a placebo, but those differences were not statistically significant.

Currently, there is no recommendation for the use of vitamin E or selenium as a chemoprevention agent.

A number of other agents are being investigated as to whether they can be useful for prostate cancer prevention. These include statins, which are drugs that lower harmful cholesterol levels, and metformin, which is used in patients with diabetes.

Contrary to popular claims, we do not have enough scientific evidence that indicates vitamin and dietary supplements prevent cancer. Several vitamins and minerals have also been studied, including vitamin B6, vitamin B12, vitamin D, beta carotene, and folic acid, but they have not been shown to lower the risk of cancer.

> **NOTE to PATIENT:**
> Learn about your family medical history, including your parents, grandparents, aunts, uncles, and cousins! As discussed in Chapter 3, family medical history is one of the most important risk factors for many cancers. Construct a pedigree diagram of your family to share with your doctor.

MY JOURNEY

I've been a nonconformist all my life. When all my friends were going off to college, I got a job on a freighter and sailed all over the world, earning a ton of money and seeing places I never knew existed. When my friends got married and started having families, I started a foster home with my sister. I voted Republican, even though I'm probably the only one I know. Whatever. But when it came to having checkups, I played it straight. My family has a terrible history of cancer, and I figured it was only a matter of time before my turn came. I was right, except that I was diligent and caught it way early, while it barely had a stage assignment and well before treatment would become an issue. So while I choose to live the rest of my life decidedly out of the box, when it comes to cancer I fall right in line and play by the rules.

Mario (Bloomington, Indiana)

HPV Vaccine:
A Poster Child for Cancer Prevention

Armed with the knowledge that human papillomavirus (HPV) is the cause of a number of cancers, including cervical, vaginal, anal, and head and neck cancers, researchers have been able to move on to the next logical step. By creating a vaccine, which would prevent the infection in people exposed to it, they hoped to decrease or eliminate the risk of HPV leading to cancer.

Cancer vaccines belong to a class of substances known as biological response modifiers. These work by stimulating or restoring the immune system's ability to fight infections and disease. There are two broad types of cancer vaccines:

1. *Preventive* (prophylactic) vaccines intend to prevent cancer from developing in healthy people
2. *Treatment* (therapeutic) vaccines intend to treat an existing cancer by strengthening the body's natural immune response against the cancer. Treatment vaccines are a form of immunotherapy.

Two types of cancer preventive vaccines (human papillomavirus vaccines and hepatitis B virus vaccines) are available in the United States, and one treatment vaccine (for metastatic prostate cancer) is also available.

How Cancer-Preventive Vaccines Work

Cancer-preventive vaccines target infectious agents that cause or contribute to the development of cancer. They are similar to traditional vaccines that help prevent infectious diseases, such as measles or polio, by protecting the body against infection. Both cancer-preventive vaccines and traditional vaccines are based on antigens (markers) found on the infectious agents, which the immune system recognizes as foreign. Preventive vaccines stimulate the production of antibodies that bind to specific targeted microbes and block their ability to cause infection.

Cancer-preventive vaccines approved by the FDA are made using antigens from Hepatitis B (HBV, one cause of liver cancer) and specific types of HPV. These antigens are proteins that help make up the outer surface of the viruses. Because only part of these microbes is used, the resulting vaccines are not infectious and, therefore, cannot cause disease.

Similarly, cancer treatment vaccines are made using cancer-associated antigens or modified versions of them. Antigens that have been used thus far include proteins, carbohydrates (sugars), glycoproteins or glycopeptides (carbohydrate-protein combinations), and gangliosides (carbohydrate-lipid combinations).

Before any vaccine is licensed, the FDA must conclude that it is both safe and effective. Vaccines intended to prevent or treat cancer appear to have safety profiles comparable to those of other vaccines. However, the side effects of cancer vaccines can vary among vaccine formulations—and from one person to another.

The most commonly reported side effect of cancer vaccines is inflammation at the site of injection, along with a chance of redness, pain, warming of the skin, itchiness, and even a rash.

People sometimes experience flu-like symptoms after receiving a cancer vaccine, including fever, chills, weakness, dizziness, nausea or vomiting, muscle ache, fatigue, headache, and occasional breathing difficulties. Blood pressure may also be affected. These side effects, which usually last for only a short time, indicate that the body is responding to the vaccine and making an immune response, as it does when exposed to a virus.

For more information about the HPV vaccine, see Chapter 6.

Cancer Screening: A Harm-Benefit Analysis

Checking for cancer—or conditions that may become cancer—in people who have no symptoms is called screening. It can help doctors find and treat several types of cancer before they become more difficult to treat. Early detection is important because when abnormal tissue or cancer is found early, it may be easier to treat. By the time symptoms appear, cancer may have begun to spread and is harder to treat. Several screening tests can detect cancer early and thereby reduce the chance of dying from that cancer.

But it is important to note the potential risks regarding screening tests because they can present potential harmful effects along with their benefits. Some of these include:

- *Bleeding* or other health problems may occur as a result of a screening process.
- *False-positive results* indicate that cancer may be present, even though it is not. False-positive test results can cause anxiety and are usually followed by additional tests and procedures that also may be harmful.
- *False-negative results* indicate that cancer is *not* present, even though it is. These test results may provide incorrect reassurance, delaying a proper diagnosis, and may cause an individual to put off seeking medical care even if symptoms develop.

- *Overdiagnosis* is possible when a screening test correctly shows that a person has cancer, but the cancer is slow growing and would not have harmed that person in his or her lifetime. Treatment of such cancers is called overtreatment.

MY JOURNEY

No one tipped me off that managing expectations would become one of the most challenging aspects of having cancer and dealing with the crazy assortment of tests, evaluations, and decisions I had to make, often on my own, it seemed, at crazy hours of the night when the only way I could get myself to sleep was by settling in on a course of action I could accept. For me, in times of unusual—and sometimes unbearable—stress I need people to be straight and give me the goods, even if it's bad. While a sugarcoated version may seem like a nice way to go, trust me, it's worthless. How can anyone make a serious choice if no one is leveling with them?

Kerry (Lincoln, Nebraska)

Prostate Cancer Screening

The digital rectal examination (DRE) and prostate specific antigen (PSA) test have been studied to assess their usefulness as screening procedures for prostate cancer. DRE is an examination of the rectum. The doctor or nurse inserts a lubricated, gloved finger into the rectum and feels the prostate through the rectal wall. The test lasts about ten to fifteen seconds and checks for the size, firmness, and texture of the prostate, any hard areas, lumps, or growth spreading beyond the prostate, as well as any pain caused by touching or pressing the prostate.

PSA is a protein produced by cells of the prostate gland. The blood test measures the PSA level. A laboratory analyzes the sample. The results are usually reported as nanograms of PSA per milliliter (ng/mL) of blood, and in men with prostate cancer, the PSA level is often elevated.

The FDA first approved this test in 1986 to monitor the progression of prostate cancer in men who had already been diagnosed. In 1994, the FDA approved the use of the PSA test in conjunction with a DRE to test asymptomatic men for prostate cancer.

Until recently, many doctors and professional organizations encouraged yearly PSA screening for men, beginning at age fifty. Some recommended that men at a higher risk of prostate cancer, including African American men and those whose father or brother had prostate cancer, begin screening at age forty or forty-five. However, as more is learned about both the benefits and harms of prostate cancer screening, a number of organizations, including the U.S. Preventive Services Task Force (USPSTF), have begun to caution against routine population screening.

Several randomized trials of prostate cancer screening have been carried out. One of the largest is the Prostate, Lung, Colorectal, and Ovarian (PLCO) Cancer Screening Trial. The study, conducted by the National Cancer Institute, was designed to determine whether certain screening tests can help reduce the numbers of deaths from several common cancers.

In the prostate portion of the trial, the PSA test and DRE were evaluated for their ability to decrease a man's chances of dying from prostate cancer. The investigators found that men who underwent annual prostate cancer screening had a higher incidence of prostate cancer than men in the control group, but the same rate of deaths from the disease.[55]

---

55. *http://www.ncbi.nlm.nih.gov/pubmed/22228146*

Overall, the results suggest that many men who were treated for prostate cancers would not have had the disease detected in their lifetime without screening. Consequently, these men were exposed unnecessarily to the potential harms of treatment.

A second large trial, the European Randomized Study of Screening for Prostate Cancer (ERSPC), compared prostate cancer deaths in men randomly assigned to PSA-based screening or no screening. As in the PLCO, men in ERSPC who were screened for prostate cancer had a higher incidence of the disease than the others. In contrast to the PLCO, however, men who were screened had a lower rate of death from prostate cancer. The USPSTF points out that these results were "heavily influenced by the results of two countries, and five of the seven countries reporting results did not find a statistically significant reduction."[56]

Routine Screening: The New Taboo

For several reasons, the USPSTF no longer recommends routine screening.

Detecting prostate cancer early may not reduce the chance of dying from prostate cancer. When used in screening, the PSA test can help detect small tumors that do not cause symptoms. Finding a small tumor, however, may not necessarily reduce a man's chance of dying from prostate cancer. Some tumors found through PSA testing grow so slowly that they are unlikely to threaten a man's life. Detecting tumors that are not life threatening is called overdiagnosis, and treating these tumors is called overtreatment.

Overtreatment exposes men unnecessarily to the potential complications and harmful side effects of treatments for early prostate

---

56. *http://www.uspreventiveservicestaskforce.org/Page/Document/RecommendationStatementFinal/ prostate-cancer-screening*

cancer, including surgery and radiation therapy. The side effects of these treatments include urinary incontinence (an inability to control urine flow), problems with bowel function, erectile dysfunction (loss of erections or an inability to have and maintain sexual intercourse), and infection. In addition, as discussed in Chapters 8 and 9, treatments for cancer, such as surgery, radiation, and chemotherapy, may have serious side effects.

It's also been shown that finding cancer early may not help a man who has a fast-growing or aggressive tumor that may have spread to other parts of the body before being detected.

Follow-up tests, such as a biopsy, may be used to diagnose cancer. If a PSA test is higher than normal, a biopsy of the prostate may be done. Complications from a biopsy of the prostate may include fever, pain, blood in the urine or semen, and urinary tract infection. Even if a biopsy shows no prostate cancer, a patient may worry more about developing it in the future.

False-negative test results can also occur. They may appear to be normal even though prostate cancer is present. A man who receives a false-negative test result—one that shows no cancer when there really is—may delay seeking medical care even if he has symptoms.

False-positive test results are possible, too. Screening results may appear to be abnormal even though no cancer is present. A false-positive test result—one that shows cancer when there really isn't—can cause anxiety and is usually followed by more tests, such as a biopsy, which also have risks.

The following chart summarizes the USPSTF recommendations.

You can examine the analysis of the data from the PLCO, ERSPC, and other trials in another way. For example, the USPSTF estimates that for every 1,000 men ages fifty-five to sixty-nine years who are screened every one to four years for a decade, zero to one death from prostate cancer would be avoided. They also claim that 100 to 120

U.S. Preventive Services Task Force

Screening for prostate cancer, clinical summary of U.S. Preventive Services Task Force recommendation

Population	Adult Males
Recommendation	Do not use prostate-specific antigen (PSA)-based screening for prostate cancer. **Grade: D**
Screening Tests	Contemporary recommendations for prostate cancer screening all incorporate the measurement of serum PSA levels; other methods of detection, such as digital rectal examination or ultrasonography, may be included. There is convincing evidence that PSA-based screening programs result in the detection of many cases of asymptomatic prostate cancer, and that a substantial percentage of men who have asymptomatic cancer detected by PSA screening have a tumor that either will not progress or will progress so slowly that it would have remained asymptomatic for the man's lifetime. (i.e., PSA-based screening results in considerable overdiagnosis).
Interventions	Management strategies for localized prostate cancer include watchful waiting, active surveillance, surgery, and radiation therapy. There is no consensus regarding optimal treatment.
Balance of Harms and Benefits	The reduction in prostate cancer mortality 10 to 14 years after PSA-based screening is, at most, very small, even for men in the optimal age-range of 55 to 69 years. The harms of screening include pain, fever, bleeding, infection, and transient urinary difficulties associated with prostate biopsy, psychological harm of false-positive test results, and overdiagnosis. Harms of treatment include erectile dysfunction, urinary incontinence, bowel dysfunction, and a small risk for premature death. Because of the current inability to reliably distinguish tumors that will remain indolent from those destined to be lethal, many men are being subjected to the harms of treatment for prostate cancer that will never become symptomatic. The benefits of PSA-based screening for prostate cancer do not outweigh the harms.
Relevant USPSTF Recommendations	Recommendations on screening for other types of cancer can be found at www.uspreventiveservicestaskforce.org/.

For a summary of the evidence systematically reviewed in making these recommendations, the full recommendation statement, and supporting documents, please go to www.uspreventiveservicestaskforce.org/.

men would have a false-positive test result that leads to a biopsy, and about one-third of the men who get a biopsy would experience at least moderately bothersome symptoms from the biopsy. Finally, 110 men would be diagnosed with prostate cancer. Of these, about fifty would have a complication from treatment, including erectile dysfunction in twenty-nine men, urinary incontinence in eighteen men, serious cardiovascular events in two men, deep vein thrombosis or pulmonary embolism in one man, and death due to the treatment in less than a single man.

Your doctor can advise you about your risk for prostate cancer and your need for screening tests.

—————————— MY JOURNEY ——————————

I fervently believe that we live in a world full of poisons, and that this will not abate in our lifetime, not as long as so many huge corporations continue to pollute our waters with waste and get filthy rich from all the toxic products they are selling us. Greed is the master of our universe. We are subject to its side effects, and cancer is right there at the top of the list, along with poverty and war. So as long as this remains true—and with a clear eye I can say it will be for a long, long time—we must be vigilant and protect ourselves as much as possible. That means living a tranquil life to the best of our ability, treating others with kindness and love, and taking care of ourselves by paying attention to the ongoing threat of cancer and other diseases. That means going to the doctor and being tested, because in this world of poisons in which we live, we are all at risk.

Diego (Seaside Heights, New Jersey)

Where Do We Go from Here?

Centers for Disease Control statistics show that aside from non-melanoma skin cancer, prostate cancer is the most common cancer among men in the United States. Their most recent data from 2012 shows that among men, black men had the highest rate of cancer, followed by white, Hispanic, Asian-Pacific Islander, and American Indian–Alaska Native men. While the overall rate of these cancers is declining annually at a rate between 3 and 4 percent, several studies predict that the frequency of prostate cancer cases in the United States will increase more than 50 percent in the coming decades, which is largely due to an aging population.

As efforts continue to make men's cancer screening available to everyone, especially those in underserved communities, we can take heart that the numbers are generally improving—some at a faster rate than was imagined just a few years ago.

It takes a village—patient, provider, and healthcare system—working together to make effective cancer screening programs that can achieve high screening rates. It's a question of synergy, combining better patient responsibility, innovations in technology, increased access to primary care services, community organizing, and improvements in the insurance system to create an environment that can better serve the needs of America's men and their families. There are lessons to be learned about screening programs from success stories in this country and around the world. Now is the time to urge our political and business leaders to prioritize these improvements.

KEY POINTS TO REMEMBER

✓ At its root, cancer is a disease of your DNA.

✓ Most cancers are not caused by inherited genes but by damage to your DNA that occurs in your lifetime.

✓ Knowing your family medical history, screening, and early detection will be the main tools for saving your life from cancer.

✓ Early detection is vital because when cancer is found early, it is almost always easier to treat.

✓ It is just as important to know the potential risks as well as the possible benefits when considering screening tests. Tests with high false-positive rates can expose you to unnecessary procedures.

✓ Currently, the USPSTF does not recommend routine PSA screening for all men.

✓ There is no screening test for testicular cancer.

✓ Vaccination with the human papillomavirus (HPV) vaccine is important in preventing a number of cancers, including cancer of the penis. It is most effective when given before a person is sexually active.

✓ Chemoprevention refers to the use of drugs to lower the risk of cancer or keep it from recurring.

✓ Contrary to popular claims, vitamin and dietary supplements have not been shown to prevent cancer.

What Cancer Cannot Do

Cancer is so limited . . .
It cannot cripple love.
It cannot shatter hope.
It cannot corrode faith.
It cannot eat away peace.
It cannot destroy confidence.
It cannot kill friendship.
It cannot shut out memories.
It cannot silence courage.
It cannot reduce eternal life.

It cannot quench the spirit.

11

EMBRACING THE TWENTY-FIRST CENTURY: Changing Definitions and the Future of Cancer

Cancer is a word, not a sentence.

—John Diamond, *The Times*/BBC,
author, *C: Because Cowards Get Cancer Too . . .*

The Times They Are a-Changin'

The Chief Medical Officer of the American Cancer Society, Dr. Otis Brawley, has declared that "We need a twenty-first century definition of cancer instead of a nineteenth century definition, which is what we've been using." We now understand that cancer is not a singular disease but hundreds of different diseases, all resulting from specific "misprints" (mutations) in our DNA, which affect everyone differently. In fact, not all of the conditions we traditionally define as cancer will progress to metastases and death. For a growing number of cancers, they will simply be viewed as another chronic illness, like type 2 diabetes or high blood pressure. Treatments based on precision diagnosis and personalized treatment will *manage* the cancer instead of trying to destroy it with harsh methods that have serious side effects.

In 2009, prominent surgeon Dr. Laura Esserman and her colleagues made the diagnosis that the term "cancer" is overused in labeling some conditions that are unlikely to cause harm if left untreated. Examples of such conditions include ductal carcinoma *in situ* (DCIS) of the breast and prostate cancers with Gleason scores of 6 or lower. Dr. Esserman's "prescription" was to rename these conditions IDLE (indolent lesions of epithelial origin) and not refer to them as cancer at all. In 2014, Dr. Esserman and a panel of experts assembled by the National Cancer Institute renewed this prescription to prevent over-diagnosis and over-treatment of certain "pre-cancerous" conditions.

Another vital new concept is "less is more." For example, some cancers of the head and neck, caused by human papilloma virus (HPV), have a better prognosis than similar cancers caused by TP53 gene mutations. Doctors are now "de-intensifying" treatment of patients with HPV-positive tumors, reducing the cost of treatment *and* the risk of patients suffering short- and long-term side effects. New methods for precision diagnosis of cancer will yield many additional opportunities for de-intensification of treatment.

Reimagining Diagnosis and Treatment

In the not-too-distant future, a blood test to detect many types of cancer may just be another part of your annual physical, like checking your blood sugar and cholesterol. Researchers have discovered that once cancer forms, even if it's too small to see on an X-ray or CT scan, some cancer cells leak their tumor DNA into the bloodstream.

Abundant research is currently studying whether liquid biopsies (blood tests) to detect this "circulating tumor DNA" (ctDNA) can be used for early detection of cancer, monitoring treatment responses, and early detection of recurrences or resistance to treatments.

Technologically, it's getting easier and cheaper to check large collections of genes for smoking gun mutations that indicate cancer, even for the very tiny amounts of ctDNA that tumors leak into the bloodstream.

What could this mean for patients? Could tests eventually be available for all men that can catch cancers early before they grow out of control and start producing symptoms?

A recent advance is the development of immunotherapy drugs that attack cancer cells in an entirely different way than drugs targeted at specific cancer genes. In some cancers, such as malignant melanoma and lung cancer, tumor cells are known to harbor a plethora of abnormal changes in their DNA, called a high mutational burden.

To make a long story short, these numerous DNA defects can lead to changes in the cells that make them look like foreign invaders in our immune systems. But cancer cells are devious and usually find ways to escape an immune response. The new drugs called immune checkpoint inhibitors block the cancer from escaping and enable special immune cells, T-cells, to capture and kill the tumor.

Four of these new drugs are currently available and one was used in the near-miraculous cure of former President Jimmy Carter, whose malignant skin cancer had invaded both his liver and brain.

Immune checkpoint inhibitors that are currently approved by the FDA to treat cancer include:

- Ipilimumab (Yervoy), approved to treat advanced melanoma (skin cancer)

- Nivolumab (Opdivo), approved to treat advanced melanoma, some types of lung cancer, and kidney cancer
- Pembrolizumab (Keytruda), approved to treat advanced melanoma and some types of lung cancer
- Atezolizumab (Tecentriq), to treat advanced bladder cancer after other treatments have failed

In fact, this "immune checkpoint" approach is so promising that pharmaceutical companies are investing large amounts of money and research into developing more drugs of this type. They are also testing how these existing drugs can be used to treat more types of cancer, including male breast cancer (Chapter 5).

───────────── MY JOURNEY ─────────────

I am not a doctor. I do not have cancer. But I am sure that love can help to cure it. Excuse me that I cannot produce any scientific evidence for this, but I have seen it work when my mother was diagnosed. At first, everyone in our house was silent, as if we might say the wrong thing simply by opening our mouths. Then I saw my father so tenderly holding my mother's hand and my sister stroking her hair. As I watched, I could not only see the smile emerging on my mother's face, I could feel her healing right in front of me! I knew in that moment that her cure could not come only from her doctors and the treatments they prescribed. It was up to us, and her, to coax away the cancer with love—with a fierce, unbending song of positivity.

That's what we did. We eliminated any shred of negativity from our house and replaced it with love, every minute of every day. Every painful moment my mother felt was accompanied by a loving touch, a terrible joke, and a soothing bit of music. Every moment of fear was met with a lovely dream to look forward to. This became our normal way to live, and when my mother was supposed to feel sick from treatment, she began to stabilize. When her doctors expected her to suffer, she did not. All the love penetrated every one of her cells, until she began to love herself in ways I had never before witnessed. I believe this gave her strength and a resolve she may not have had before, and this carried her, too, along with our love.

Now, a few years later, my mother is cancer-free and volunteering at the center, encouraging patients and doctors and nurses, anyone she comes into contact with, to embrace the power of love. I am no doctor, but I do know that love can do magic. It can even cure cancer.

Jamie (Hartford, Connecticut)

Do We Need a "Moonshot" to Cure Cancer? and Why Now?

In President Obama's January 2016 State of the Union address, he called for a new "moonshot" to cure cancer—a program to be led by Vice President Joe Biden, whose son died of brain cancer in May 2015. "This is personal for me," Biden told *AARP The Magazine* in March 2016. "But this is personal for just about every American and millions around the world."

As we've explained throughout the book, tremendous advances in cancer research and treatment have been made since 2001. In fact, during these past fifteen years, so many advances have accumulated that we have now reached a critical mass of knowledge and experience, placing us on the brink of transforming cancer into a manageable illness, even if we might not be able to completely cure it in all cases.

This accumulated knowledge base is a launching pad for an attack on cancer so broad and meaningful that nothing like it has been seen since President Nixon first declared the War on Cancer forty-five years ago, in 1971.

Specific plans for this concentrated push to cure cancer are still being drawn up as we complete this book, but allow us to share our vision of what we would like the goals of this cancer moonshot to be.

Goal #1: Better Education and New Tools for Training of Healthcare Professionals

Advances in cancer diagnosis and treatment have been so rapid that most doctors never learn about them in medical school. The result is that even currently available drugs and diagnostics are being underutilized or utilized improperly. According to a March 2015 story in *Time*, fewer than 5 percent of the 1.6 million people diagnosed with cancer each year in the United States have access to cancer DNA testing. One important reason is that many doctors don't understand the technology and how best to use it.

The March 2013 issue of *The Oprah Magazine* said, "DNA research has led to cutting-edge breakthroughs in how we detect cancer risk. But when doctors can't keep up with the science, the results can be perilous."

As the *New York Times* reported earlier this year, "The genetic data is there, but in many cases, doctors do not know what to do with it."[57]

Goal #2: Applied Research in the Optimal Use of Currently Available Therapies

At the present time, about sixty targeted drugs and immunotherapies have been approved by the FDA for the treatment of various types of cancer. Traditionally, a new cancer drug is approved to treat only one type of cancer but is later found to be useful for other cancer types, based on underlying genetic similarities among diverse tumor types. Remember imatinib (Gleevec) from Chapter 1? This drug was

---

57. Gina Kolata, "When Gene Tests for Breast Cancer Reveal Grim Data but No Guidance," *New York Times*, March 11, 2016.

originally approved (indicated) in 2001 to treat one relatively uncommon blood cancer called CML. But now, fifteen years later, the indications of imatinib have expanded to at least eight different types of cancers or cancer-like conditions.

Another example is how and when to use individual drugs or combinations and how to sequence these therapies at different times. For example, the malignant skin cancer melanoma could be successfully treated with a single drug (monotherapy) called vemurafenib (Zelboraf), but most patients developed resistance to treatment and their cancers came back after a year. Doctors discovered that combination therapy with two different drugs (dabrafenib [Tafinlar] and trametinib [Mekinist]) that attack different weak points in the tumor at the same time lead to more durable responses—meaning the tumors don't come back as quickly, or at all. Things are changing once again in the treatment of melanoma patients, with many doctors treating first with immunotherapies and saving the gene-targeted drugs to be used later, if necessary.

Goal #3: Development of New Services Unique to Long-Term Survivors

If many cancers really do become manageable chronic illnesses like high blood pressure or diabetes, patients will need new types of services and resources to help with special challenges, such as coping with potential long-term side effects or after effects of treatment (Chapter 8).

Goal #4: Pursuit of New Biomedical Research Opportunities

In the May 19, 2016 issue of *The New England Journal of Medicine*, Dr. Douglas Lowy, Director of the National Cancer Institute, and Dr. Francis Collins, Director of the National Institutes of Health, published a plan for the Cancer Moonshot Program. It promised that by the end of the summer of 2016, a Blue Ribbon Panel would provide recommendations to the National Cancer Advisory Board on the most exceptional opportunities in cancer research. These are likely to include early detection technologies, cancer vaccines and immunotherapies, unique aspects of childhood cancers and data sharing intended to break down barriers between public and private research organizations.

Challenges for Patients and Society

We must mention one fundamental factor that needs to be a priority of President Obama's moonshot. In fact, it may be the only way that any of these potential advances can come to fruition, saving millions of people from suffering unnecessarily from cancer.

That is the study of oncoeconomics—the economics of cancer care.

All of the exciting developments that we've talked about create formidable economic challenges for society. The first reason is that patients will live much longer but require treatment and new services for the rest of their lives. Second, a single targeted cancer drug or immunotherapy can cost thousands of dollars per month. If a new standard of care involves combinations of drugs that have to be taken for years, the potential costs become staggering.

Together, we all need to figure out the best ways to tackle cancer and save our own lives. As we've mentioned repeatedly, prevention needs to come first, and that is a team effort that needs all of us to participate.

KEY POINTS TO REMEMBER

✓ We need a twenty-first-century definition of cancer instead of a nineteenth-century definition.

✓ During the past fifteen years, so many advances have been made that we have now reached a critical mass of knowledge and experience that allows us to reimagine cancer as a manageable illness.

✓ Some diseases we used to call cancer have been "downgraded" with less frightening names.

✓ Some cancer treatments are being de-intensified.

✓ In the not-too-distant future, a blood test to detect many types of cancer may just be another part of your annual physical exam.

✓ Oncoeconomics refers to the economics of cancer care.

✓ Prevention needs to come first, and that is a team effort that needs all of us to participate.

What Cancer Cannot Do

Cancer is so limited . . .
It cannot cripple love.
It cannot shatter hope.
It cannot corrode faith.
It cannot eat away peace.
It cannot destroy confidence.
It cannot kill friendship.
It cannot shut out memories.
It cannot silence courage.
It cannot reduce eternal life.
It cannot quench the spirit.

—Author unknown

About the Authors

Mark S. Boguski, MD, PhD, FCAP

Dr. Mark S. Boguski is the founder and Chief Medical Officer of Precision Medicine Network, Inc.

He has served on the faculites at Harvard Medical School and Beth Israel Deaconess Medical Center, the Johns Hopkins University School of Medicine, the Fred Hutchinson Cancer Research Center and the U.S. National Institutes of Health. He is a past faculty member of the Molecular Biology in Clinical Oncology workshop at the American Association for Cancer Research.

Dr. Boguski has also served as Vice President of the Novartis Institute for Biomedical Research and as the founding Director of the Paul Allen Institute for Brain Science. He has been an advisor and consultant to numerous medical research organizations, including the Merck Genome Research Institute, the Genetics Advisory Group for the Wellcome Trust, and the Howard Hughes Medical Institute.

Dr. Boguski has received the Regents' Award from the National Library of Medicine and the Director's Award from the National Institutes of Health. He is an elected member of the National Academy of Medicine, a Fellow of the College of American Pathologists, and a Fellow of the American College of Medical Informatics, as well as former reviewing editor for *Science* magazine and past Editor-in-Chief of the journal of *Genomics*.

Dr. Boguski received his BA from the Johns Hopkins University and an MD and PhD from the Medical Scientist Training Program at Washington University School of Medicine.

Michele R. Berman, MD

Michele Berman, MD, is a graduate of the Washington University School of Medicine in St. Louis, Missouri, and completed her residency in Pediatrics at Children's Hospital in St. Louis. She served as Staff Pediatrician at DePaul Hospital in Bridgeton, Missouri, and as Clinical Instructor at Georgetown University and George Washington University in Washington, DC. She practiced general pediatrics in a private practice on Capitol Hill for twelve years. She also served on courtesy or active staff at other Washington-area medical facilities, including Children's Hospital National Medical Center, Columbia Hospital for Women, Holy Cross Hospital, and Shady Grove Adventist Hospital.

During her sixteen years in primary care medical practice, Dr. Berman interacted with thousands of "consumers," having to explain to them complex medical concepts in layperson's terms. This experience was supplemented and extended through her monthly consumer advice column in *Washington Parent Magazine*.

In 1997, she established one of the first private practice websites in the country—*ThePediatricCenter.com*—in Washington, DC, and Bethesda, Maryland. This site served as an additional communication channel for the consumer health information in her *Washington Parent* articles, and it employed rudimentary social networking features such as patients submitting their school artwork to be featured on the site.

In late 2008, Dr. Berman founded *Celebrity Diagnosis* to take her medical journalism to Web 2.0 communications. This work has been recognized by several local and national media organizations, such as the *Wall Street Journal*, the *Boston Globe*, Fox25 News and WCVB News in Boston, New England Cable News, and the *San Diego Union-Tribune*. Since January 2009, she has written 200 stories about cancer and has written or coauthored over 1,000 articles about other diseases, medical conditions, and consumer health topics.

Her tweets on Twitter and posts on Facebook are followed by many, including consumers, physicians, nurses, psychologists, nutritionists, medical writers, social media marketing experts, women's magazines, the Pew Internet and American Life Project, the Robert Wood Johnson Foundation, the Medicine and Health editor for *USA Today* (Liz Szabo), and *American Medical News*.

Dr. Berman is a Fellow of the American Academy of Pediatrics, a former Member of the Medical Society of the District of Columbia and the Montgomery County Medical Society. Her awards include *Phi Beta Kappa* from Johns Hopkins University and *Omicron Delta Kappa* from Johns Hopkins University's National Leadership Society.

HealthPlus Health Plan named her Outstanding Primary Care Physician and she has been cited by *Washingtonian Magazine* as an Outstanding Washington Physician.

David Tabatsky

David Tabatsky is a writer, editor, teacher, director and performing artist. He received his BA in Communications and an MA in Theatre Education, both from Adelphi University.

David is the author of *Write for Life: Communicating Your Way Through Cancer* and coauthor of *The Cancer Book: 101 Stories of Courage, Support and Love* and editor of Elizabeth Bayer's *It's Just a Word*, both published by Chicken Soup for the Soul Publishing in 2009. He is the coauthor, with Bruce Kluger, of *Dear President Obama: Letters of Hope from Children Across America* also published in 2009. David wrote *The Boy Behind the Door: How Salomon Kool Escaped the Nazis* (2009). With Dr. Mark Banschick, David coauthored *The Intelligent Divorce*—Books One and Two (2009 and 2010, respectively) and *The Wright Choice: Your Family's Guide to Healthy Eating, Modern Fitness and Saving Money* (2011), with Dr. Randy Wright. David was the consulting editor for Marlo Thomas and her *New York Times* bestseller *The Right Words at the Right Time, Volume 2: Your Turn* (2006). He has published two editions of *What's Cool Berlin* a comic travel guide to Germany's capital, and has written for *The Forward, Parenting,* and *Sesame Street Parent*, among others.

David has worked professionally in theater and circus as an actor, clown, and juggler, at New York City's Lincoln Center, Radio City Music Hall, the Beacon Theatre and throughout the United States and Europe, most notably at the Chamäleon in Berlin, New End Theatre in London, Folies Pigalle in Paris, and the Edinburgh Fringe Festival, where *The Stage* wrote, "He is a supremely skillful performer and a fine actor, reaching levels no other comics have matched at this Fringe." David also directed *Kinderzirkus Taborka* at the renowned Tempodrom in Berlin.

David has taught theater and circus arts for the American School of London, die Etage in Berlin, the Big Apple Circus School, The United Nations International School, and the Cathedral of St. John the Divine. He served on the theater faculty at Adelphi University and The Cooper Union and as a teaching artist for the Henry Street Settlement with a focus on special education. He has taught circus arts at Sunrise Day Camp, America's only dedicated day camp for children with cancer and their siblings.

David teaches writing and communication workshops and speaks on these subjects at cancer centers through the United States.

Please visit *www.tabatsky.com* and *www.writeforlife.info*.

About Celebrity Diagnosis

Celebrity Diagnosis and Celebrity Diagnosis Professional Edition have been nominated for the annual medGadget Weblog Award in the categories of Best Medical Blog and Best New Medical Blog.

Please visit *www.celebritydiagnosis.com*.

For more information, including resources and recommended reading, please visit: *www.reimaginingcancer.com*.

About *Reimagining Women's Cancers*

Reimagining Women's Cancers, the patient-friendly companion book in the *Reimagining Cancer* series, covers breast, ovarian, vaginal/vulvar, endometrial/uterine, and cervical cancers. For example, the chapter on breast cancer begins with a view of basic anatomy, an overview of how we view breast cancer today, signs, symptoms, and diagnosis, as well as scientific information on mammogram guidelines and ultrasound.

The book also includes a comprehensive survey of treatments, breast reconstruction, prevention, and short- and long-term forecasts. Woven throughout are celebrity stories, both medical and anecdotal, from women, including Angelina Jolie, Joan Lunden, Melissa Etheridge, Sandra Lee, Rita Wilson, Christina Applegate, and Suzanne Somers, as well as personal anecdotes from patients around the country.

For the more than 354,000 women diagnosed each year in the Unites States with cancer of the breast, ovaries, endometrium, uterus, and cervix, as well as for the loved ones and medical professionals who care for them, *Reimagining Women's Cancers* is for you.

We must try to contribute joy to the world.
That is true no matter what our problems,
our health, our circumstances.
We must try.
I didn't always know this and I am happy
I lived long enough to find it out.

—Roger Ebert

Index